Gout Relief

Live Your Life Without Pain and Distress With Natural Remedies

(Natural and Effective Remedies to Get Rid of Gout Problem)

Dennis Brewer

Published By **Chris David**

Dennis Brewer

Gout Relief: Live Your Life Without Pain and Distress With Natural Remedies (Natural and Effective Remedies to Get Rid of Gout Problem)

ISBN   978-1-998901-69-2

Legal & Disclaimer

Table of Contents

Chapter 1: Understanding What Gout Is

To endure a certain situation or issue it is essential to be aware of the. Gout is one of these conditions. Knowing it is the way towards being able manage it and be able to live with it.

Perhaps the most well-known type of arthritis or joint inflammation, gout , also known as Gouty arthritis has a long and illustrious background with the first depictions of it dating way back to the 5th century B.C. In fact, gout has been called "the disease of kings" due to its connection with rich food and alcohol consumption. In 2011, however, we learned that gout does not choose who it will affect by the status of their finances. Instead, it's diagnosed with the digestion of uric acid. Gout is a severe and painful form of arthritis, which is included within a class of arthropathies called the "crystalline arthritis.' Gout is caused due to a pronounced inflammation reaction to uric acid crystals that occur when there is hyperuricemia (high levels of uric acid in blood).

Gout is an joint inflammation that occurs in people with high levels uric acid in their blood. The acid can cause needle-like crystals develop in joints and trigger sudden, severe instances of delicacy, pain, hotness, redness, and swelling.

The supersaturation of uric acids causes crystal aggregation and release from tissues and joints in which our immune system reacts. Tophi uric acid (which is present in tophaceous Gout) manifest as hard, granular knobs beneath the skin. They can cause a lot of destruction and discomfort.

The link between gout and the uric acid is well-known from the beginning of the nineteenth century but it's the dramatic improvements in our understanding of the adroit uric acid homeostasis that have led to the an effective treatment of Gout. Gout is still one of the most manageable forms of arthritis.

History of Gout

The term "gout" was at first used to describe gout by Randolphus of Bocking at around 1200 AD. The word "gout" is derived via"gutta," the Latin word gutta which means "a drop" (of liquid). According to the Oxford English Dictionary, this originates from humorism as well as "the notion of the 'dropping' of a morbid material from the blood in and around the joints."

Gout is known since the beginning of time. In fact, it was referred to by "the king of diseases and the disease of kings" or "rich man's disease."

The first recorded evidence of this ailment comes from Egypt around 2,600 BC in a description of joint inflammation that affected the massive toe. In the Greek doctor Hippocrates about 400 BC commented on the condition in his Axioms in which he noted the absence of it in eunuchs as well as premenopausal women. Aulus Cornelius Celsus described the relationship it shares with drinking, late-onset women and the related kidney issues. He said that the thickness of urinary dregs, of which are white, indicates that inflammation and agony is possible to detect in the region around the joint. It is important to get found in the vicinity of joints. He also discussed joint pain in the feet and hands and the way they can occur for those suffering from the disease. He also suggested that the disease rarely affected prepubescent and eunuchs as well as women (in the rare exception of who are menopausal). He also believed that the people who managed to stay clear of this illness have done so by avoiding red food, alcohol and beers.

in 1683 Thomas Sydenham, an English doctor, described its prevalence during the first hours of morning, and the preference of men who are older and more wealthy. Sydenham said that patients suffering from gout generally usually elderly men or those who have consumed themselves in youth that they have accelerated the process of aging unintentionally. Of these sexually sexy traits, none more prevalent than the untimely and extravagant indulgence in red meat as well as other harmful foods. As per his research, if you indulge on these kinds of foods is when gout strikes. According to his account, the patient eats hay and sleeps in good health. About two in the early morning, he's shaken by severe pain in his big toe (and at times, but seldom in the lower leg, heel or the instep). The pain is similar to the one you feel when an ankle joint had been dislocated . Some areas of the joint feel as if cold water has been sprinkled over the joint. The next thing that occurs is a fever that manifests as shaking and chills. In his article, Sydenham states that for the patient who is suffering from a sleep disorder, the nights will be with restlessness, pain as well as a tendency to turn the affected body and shifting the sleeping position. The movements result in additional pain for the body.

The most prominent person who previously described gout, or had an opinion about gout which accurately reflects the reality of its relationship to uric acid can be traced to one of the Dutch research scientist Antonie van Leeuwenhoek, who sketched the tiny appearance of the urate crystals in 1679. Also, in 1848 English medical doctor Alfred Garrod discovered a high concentration of uric acid within the blood as a cause for gout.

What Are The Phases of Gout?

There are several types of Gout. There are several phases of

Phase one Hyperuricemia that is symptomatic

Asymptomatic hyperuricemia occurs during the time prior to the onset of gout. There are no signs however blood uric acid levels are elevated, and crystals are beginning to form within the joint.

Phase two Two: Gout attack

A severe gout attack, or Gout attack occurs whenever something (for instance an evening of drinking) causes uric acid levels to rise or shakes the crystals that are formed in joints and triggers the attack. The subsequent inflammation and pain typically begin at night and then rise over the following 8 to 12 hours. The symptoms subside after some days and are likely to disappear within 7-10 days. Some people do not experience another attack, however, the majority of those who suffer from Gout attack will experience another one within a year. The majority of people 84% could be afflicted with another attack in three years.

Phase three Gout interval

This is when there are fewer attacks. Despite the fact that there's no pain but the gout isn't totally gone. A mild aggravation can still cause damage to joints. This is a great time to treat gout with significant lifestyle changes and medication to avoid the possibility of recurring attacks or to treat chronic gout.

Fourth phase Four: Chronic gout

Chronic gout can be seen in people suffering from gout, whose uric acid levels remain high throughout the years. Attacks are more frequent and the pain might not go away as quickly as quickly as it used to. The joint may be damaged and cause the development of disability. With proper treatment and management the condition can be prevented.

5. Chronic tophaceous Gout

Gout with constant tophaceous inflammation is the most weakened form of Gout. It is possible that the last injury has occurred in joints or the kidneys. Patients can suffer from the negative effects of chronic arthritis. They can also form tophi, huge fragments of the urate crystal in cooler areas in the body. such as joints on the fingers.

It will take a long time without treatment to reach the stage of chronic Gout, which is about 10 years. It is nearly impossible for a patient to receive proper treatment will progress to this stage.

Who will be in the most danger?

Gout is a common occurrence in the same proportion of adults. This means that it affects thousands of people throughout the globe.

Risk Factors For Gout

Biology: Your genetics could put you at risk of developing gout. If your relatives suffer from Gout, you'll be prone to get it.

Other health conditions: High cholesterol levels or heart diseases diabetes, hypertension, and other conditions could increase your chance of developing gout.

Prescription drugs: Although they can be beneficial in treating your condition, certain drugs could put you at higher risk of getting Gout. Diuretic prescriptions prescribed to treat hypertension may increase the levels of uric acid; as are a number of medications that hinder the performance in the body's immune system for patients suffering from psoriasis as well as rheumatoid arthritis . transplant recipients.

Age and Sex: Gout is more typical for males than females until the age of 60. Experts believe that the regular release of estrogen helps women at this point.

Diet Consuming red meats and shellfish increase the chances of getting gout.

Liquor: For the majority of people, drinking more than two drinks of alcohol or two drinks a day can make it more likely to develop developing gout.

Soft drinks: Fructose found in soft drinks that are sweet has in recent times been identified as the cause the increase the chance of developing Gout.

Obesity: Heavy and obese people are more at risk of developing gout and generally experience it earlier than people who are normal weight.

Myths Associated With Gout

Ask anyone who has ever suffered from gout, and the primary issue they will mention is how challenging living with it is, and how often it's been misinterpreted.

Gout is a terribly painful kind of arthritis that can be experienced by anyone. It's caused by high levels of uric acid present in the blood result in crystals of urate that form within joints. If your body makes excessive amounts of uric acids or fails to get rid of uric acids in the right way it is possible to experience gout attacks. Because kidneys are the conduit for releasing urine containing uric acid those suffering from kidney disease will likely to experience an increase in crystals of urate, and as a result and Gout is a common condition.

Gout can strike at any time often, and can be accompanied by extreme attacks, referred to as flare-ups. In the event of a flare-up with gout it is possible to experience severe swelling, pain as well as redness and swelling in joints. Gout flare-ups are extremely stressful and can be difficult to manage. This condition can affect many aspects of your routine, including work relaxing or family time.

Unfortunately, a lot often Gout isn't given any attention to, and most of the time, patients are blamed for their condition. Here are some commonly held beliefs about gout. They are accompanied by truths.

Myths: Gout can be found in a small percentage of people.

The truth is that gout is a common occurrence Many people in the world suffer from gout and the number is increasing. Gout is one of the popular type of arthritis among men who are over forty years of age.

The Myth Gout is the name given to a person's disease.

The truth is that humans of all ages are susceptible to Gout. Despite the fact that males tend to be more times more likely to develop Gout, the rates of gout are generally get worse after 60 for women, as the onset of gout is generally following menopausal.

Myth: Just obese and overweight individuals get gout.

Realities: People of all sizes may suffer from Gout. In spite of the fact people who weigh more have a greater chance of developing gout, it is also common for those with other medical issues such as diabetes, high cholesterol levels hypertension, kidney disease.

The myth: Gout just affects the big toe.

Reality: The toe of the big is the most popular place where gout attacks are likely to be experienced, and a lot of people are experiencing their first gout attacks within their toes. However, gout can happen across all joints of the body, such as the knees, elbows and hands and lower legs. When people suffer from chronic gout several joint joints suffer from the condition.

The Myth of Gout always leaves you without an effective treatment

The reality: Signs that are gout-related generally disappear within a few days. However, this doesn't mean that gout isn't evident. Even if you're not feeling any side effects, urate crystals within the body could cause chronic medical problems like kidney and joint pain.

Myth: I need to do is be careful about certain things to not suffer from Gout.

Realistically, there could be certain foods that you need to stay away from if you're susceptible to gout. Additionally, certain food items can reduce levels of urinary acids within your body. However, diet alone isn't a fix. People with gout who adhere to a strict diet might, in any event require medication to stop attacks with gout. This is done by reducing the level of uric acid within their bodies.

Issues Arising From Having Gout

For this portion of the chapter, I conducted some research and talked to certain people in order to give you a clear idea of what it's like to be living with gout prior to moving into the treatment options and preventive measures can be taken. As part of the research I spoke to a few people about their experiences and all names mentioned in this section aren't the names that were originally used by the people who participated because although consent was given to incorporate their responses however, it was not given permission to use their names as they are.

The total impact on life

Despite the fact that gout-related issues significantly impact the daily lives of many people However, some thought that gout didn't had any impact on their lives in any way. They felt that way as they could easily spot and treat gout attacks, and also were able to reduce the impact of gout on their daily life.

Many people believed that gout was debilitating and that they had to sit and wait until the pain eased before returning to normal living. People who suffered from chronic attacks, and who had them periodically, believed that gout was affecting them throughout the day since they were constantly thinking about it, even when they weren't having an attack. Some people felt that it affected them for a short period during attacks.

In essence, it is true that the experiences of people are different.

Matt is prone to recurring severe attacks. Matt said that he lived an 'exciting life' prior to the onset of gout, and it has greatly affected him. However, Nathaniel however, contrary to what he said believes that gout is not a major part to his existence.

Andre says that his rheumatologist assured him that the gout issue could be managed to ensure that it did not affect his life style. Andre was pleased to learn that taking preventive medicine helped achieve this.

David declares that he was forced be able to place his own life on hold' whenever there was an attack.

Asher thinks that his second assault was uncomfortable due to how it impacted his mobility and quality of life to a great degree.

Bernice believes that many people don't realize the impact that gout can impact on all aspects of people's lives. She acknowledged that, as it's not a dangerous condition, people often minimize the severity and how weakening it can be.

Exercises and other errands

There were a variety of issues for people depending on the place their attacks took place. Making use of knives and forks was painful for Philip after he suffered an attack in his hands. Billy was unable to get his bed ready. Ian tried to carry all of his normal chores and activities even when he was having an attack, but he claimed it took him longer to accomplish things such as spreading out the laundry that had been washed. A lot of people reported that it was difficult to go to the bathroom with attacks on their lower legs, feet or knees. In one instance, Jane required assistance to take her bath.

Elle often is unable to get money or card out of the purse when she's out shopping.

Joint injuries from long hauls has made normal tasks difficult for a few people. Henry discovered it difficult to remove the caps from milk bottles made of plastic because the caps were too difficult to grasp.

Emotions, thoughts and states of mind

A lot of people I talked with who were discussing gout and how it affected their mental state or the way they felt. The discomfort, along with the restrictions it imposed on their lives, caused people feel hopeless uneasy or 'tender"confused," 'bad-tempered anger and annoyed.' The occasional bout of gout can make Lois feel depressed disoriented and 'dormant due to its fact that it restricts her public appearances and activities to a certain degree. Jane and other individuals reported that suffering from the condition brought them down or crying. A person thought that having gout was "frightening due to the crippling effect it might be causing.

When an attack occurs, Brenda finds it baffling that she's feeling well until she gets up and places pressure over her joint.

Some people thought about the possibility of gout every day and was worried about when they'd be next to suffer from an attack. Some didn't think about it even if they believed that their daily treatment had prevented from suffering attacks. Joe is still anxious about getting another attack, despite that he didn't have one in quite a time. For Michael this is a concern that always lurks in an idyll in his head. There were some who worried that they could do or eat something that could result in an attack. Some people were worried about getting warnings in the event that they fell short on their daily precaution tablets (for instance, allopurinol) or didn't take one.

Following the change according to an assessment, Philip believes that he's back to living life like normal.'

In the absence of an attack Henry recognized how ill the gout afflicted him before. People he hadn't observed for a while commented on how good his appearance was. Some people were grateful that gout was an illness that was only affecting it once or twice.

Some people were embarrassed by gout. However, some were constantly irritated because it is often viewed as a condition that is only affecting older people or males. Ian thought that a small number of people may be reluctant to get a diagnosis of gout due to their perceptions about the disease. Some people were also annoyed by others slamming Gout, despite the fact that it is, as Henry declared, "It's funny to everyone, with the only exception being the person who is in a twirl'

Sally is of the opinion that a large number of people believe that gout is unimportant, but they don't realize the pain it causes.

Some people did not feel embarrassed by having gout, however, they were embarrassed due to the impact it caused their physical movement. Ian was somewhat humiliated due to the fact that his knee was swollen and he couldn't help others in the way he normally would normally. Eddie felt it was embarrassing while he was with friends and had to struggle to get to the bathroom because of an attack on his knee.

Kelly does not feel embarrassed about the condition of gout. Kelly thinks it's simply an additional thing.'

-Sleeping

The severe pain and suffering of attacks prevented many from resting comfortably or even in any way. Sam found that not sleeping comfortably affected her mood and also increased her pain. A few people complained it difficult to settle into bed especially due to how they could not endure having sheets of bed covering their joint. Joe tried lying down with his leg a few inches off the his bed. Some people put cushions or other items on the opposite side of their joint to prevent the spreads from hitting the joint. Some people believed that it was more difficult to adjust to pain when they were sleeping because they had nothing other to do.

Anita stated that it was difficult to fall asleep in the midst of an attack. The duvet was too uncomfortable touching her foot. She also said that turning around also made her feel pain.

Some people found sitting or lying in a comfortable chair more enjoyable. They often tried their hand at watching or sat on the couch in front of the TV to distract themselves from pain and suffering. Some people moved away from their rooms to avoid causing a disturbance for others in the family who were trying to fall asleep. Some couldn't even get in their bed after an argument.

If you think you have goutissues, talk to your physician or your primary care physician about the symptoms and signs you're experiencing. If you suffer from Gout and you are experiencing symptoms, speak to your physician about the available treatment options. It is possible to get the referral of a rheumatologist or arthritis specialist, who has considerable time with patients that suffer from Gout.

Chapter 2: Symptoms Of Gout

You can be assured that number of people suffering from gout will have just one severe Gout attack during their lifetime. When you suffer from a severe Gout attack, the symptoms will disappear in a couple of days, and you might not experience another attack.

For certain people suffering from gout, it is an ongoing and persistent disease. For these individuals, it is possible to have repeated Gout attacks, and the attacks typically are more prolonged that the first attack. Patients who have recurring attacks of gout can suffer from persistent or continuous gout that will likely suffer joint damage. They'll require medication for a prolonged period both for treatment of gout as well as to stop gout attacks.

Because each person is unique and unique and it's not easy to predict when a gout-related attack might occur, it is essential to be aware of the warning signs of a gout attack especially if you suffer from chronic gout. This chapter will help you understand how to spot signs of a approaching gout attack and will also provide common signs of chronic gout.

The most basic symptoms of an attack of gout.

As previously mentioned, pain and inflammation are among the most well-known signs of an attack of gout. Gout-related agony can be seen again depicted as a intense, throbbing, and beating. The discomfort generally occurs suddenly. It could wake you up at any time during your night or be experiencing it prior to anything else as you get up in the early morning.

If you experience an attack of gout it is a constant pain and the severity of the pain can vary during the course of the duration of the attack. Although attacks typically last between three to five days, pain will be most intense in the first 24 hours following the time when the attack began. When the pain has gone the joint, there may be unease in the joint. The discomfort can last for just a few days to about a month.

In addition to the pain In addition, you might be able to see that the joint is firm swelling hot, red, and very delicate. These are signs of inflammation.

Other than pain and inflammation In addition, there are other signs and symptoms of a gout attack that you must be looking out for.

One of these signs is when it's only one joint infected by this attack. Gout attacks are the first signs that you notice. generally, affects only one joint (typically in the large toe, lower leg or knee) however, different joints may be affected also. Gout can also be found in the insteps of your feet, as well as the points of impact and wrists, elbows, and fingers. In the event that you're suffering from multiple gout attacks the joint it affects isn't likely to change. For instance, if there's an attack of gout in your toe, if you experience an attack, it's most likely to occur in the same toe. However and as you'll learn more later when gout becomes chronic, other joints may end up being included.

Another indication that can be seen in addition to inflammation and pain is the presence of a fever. Many patients experience fevers when they suffer from gout attacks.

It is not the case that every person suffering from an attack of gout will display all the signs and symptoms for an attack. It is possible to have just three or two symptoms.

The Most Effective Method To Discover Chronic Gout

It is quite possible to experience gout-related attacks when you have chronic gout. If you suffer from chronic gout, it is possible to suffer from flares. This is a time period in which your symptoms increase. In this regard it is important to be able to discern the indicators of a gout attack , and attempt to prevent attacks.

As a general rule you can have your doctor conduct an ongoing gout test in the event that you experience at minimum two severe gout attacks in one year. Keep in mind that irritation and pain don't last forever when you suffer from chronic gout. However, the two effects appear when you are experiencing an attack of gout.

Additionally, your doctor will examine the levels of uric acid in your body. Significant levels of uric acids (higher than 12 mg/dL) could assist your physician in diagnosing chronic gout as uric acid levels are expected to be in the range of 4 to 5 mg/dL. High levels of uric acid can also cause uric acids crystals accumulate in your kidneys. This can cause kidney stones, a different sign of gout that is chronic.

Another sign for chronic gout can be the tophi. Tophi are white deposits of uric acid , which look like tiny blemishes beneath the surface of the joint that is affected. They usually develop after you've suffered from gout some time.

Furthermore, many joints could be affected by chronic gout. These joints may be damaged after a certain period of period of time if the gout condition is untreated. The range of motion may also decrease within these joint. The doctor will be able to identify the most obvious signs of joint changes that are not normal in imaging tests such as X-rays.

A sign that your chronic gout may be going to be completely out of control is different for each person. But, indications that it could be more severe than you think it is could be:

Flare-ups occur more often and last longer. After a while inflammation causes long-lasting damage to ligaments and bones.

The flare-ups can occur in a variety of places in your body. About half of people with gout will experience their first attack in the joint that is at the base of the large toe. As the gout condition gets worse, it could occur at various joints, such as the knee and the lower leg.

Bumps start to develop under the skin . Uric acid crystals can start to accumulate in the delicate tissues, forming protrusions, also known as tophi. They are typically found on fingers, hands elbows, ears, and fingers. But, they could appear on any area on the human body.

Kidney problems. Your kidneys constantly eliminate the uric acid that is in your body. But, as you may imagine the amount of it may also cause harm to your organs. Gout-related kidney issues (and indications that gout is becoming worse) are kidney stones as well as kidney failure.

What do you do if you suffer from gout symptoms?

If you experience any indications of gout, such as sudden painful, gnarly pain in your joints, talk to your physician. While a severe gout attack can go away by itself, regardless of whether you take action, treating gout not treated will eventually cause progressively severe joint damage and pain. Recognizing the symptoms and signs of a gout attack may help you avoid the possibility of recurring attacks.

Chapter 3: Complications Associated With Gout

A lot of people who have an gout attack only have another attack. Some suffer from a persistent Gout-related condition or repeat attacks that occur more often after a period of. Interminable gout may lead to grave problems, especially if it is not treated.

Talk to your doctor If you are concerned about gout , or the problems it may cause.

-Effect on regular life activities

Gout attacks typically occur at night and can cause you to be woken from your beautiful sleep. In the event of persistent pain, it can prevent your from returning to the sleep you had enjoyed.

Lack of sleep can cause a variety of problems. A few of them are fatigue, fatigue that is more intense depression, mood swings and mood fluctuations.

Gout's ache and attack may also affect your ability to perform specific activities such as walking and running primary errands as well as other routine activities. Furthermore, joint injuries caused through repeated gout attacks can result in permanent incapacity.

-Tophi

Tophi are urate-containing crystals which form under the skin during cases of chronic or severe gout which is also called tophaceous Gout. The body parts that are most frequently affected by Tophi include the lower legs, feet the wrists, hands and ears.

Tophi are like bumps that feel hard beneath your skin . They're usually not painful except the occurrence of gout attacks, when they are irritated and swelling.

As tophi continue to develop and growing, they could degrade the skin and the connective tissues. This could cause damage and joint destruction.

-Joint disfigurement

If the root of the problem isn't addressed, intense attacks will become more frequent. The aggravation triggered through these assaults, such as the growth of tophi causes joint tissue damage.

Joint arthritis and joint inflammation caused by gout could trigger the disintegration of bones and ligaments, leading to total destruction in the joint.

Stones from the kidney

A similar urate crystal which is responsible for the painful adverse effects of gout could be found in kidneys too. They can cause painful kidney stones.

Urate kidney stones can interfere with kidney function.

-Kidney illnesses

Based on information gathered through the U.S. of America's National Kidney Foundation, numerous people with gout also suffer from the chronic kidney condition (CKD). It can lead to kidney failure.

However, there are conflicting opinions on whether the current kidney disease is responsible for the elevated levels of uric acid that can result in gout symptoms.

-Coronary disease

Gout is common among people suffering from hypertension, coronary arterial disease (CAD) and heart failure.

Other conditions

Other conditions that can be attributed to gout may include:

1. Cataracts or blurring of the focus of the eye. This affects the eye's ability to see.

2. Dry eye disorders

3. Uric acid crystals have been found lodged in the lung (this is however not uncommon).

Long haul view

If caught in the early stages, number of people with gout are able to go on living a normal life. If your condition has caused to gout, lowering your uric acid levels can boost joint strength and eliminate tophi.

The use of drugs and lifestyle changes can be helpful in easing the symptoms and lessening the frequency and severity of gout attacks.

Chapter 4: Getting Through A Gout Attack Bout

There's nothing more painful than a Gout attack, so if you're shook in the beginning of the morning by a joint that's fragile, swollen and glowing red You'll have to take action immediately.

This chapter I'll examine how to survive Gout attacks and what one can take to help make it easier.

Let me start with a few of the most basic actions you can do in the event of a gout attack to ease the pain of the attack as well as reduce the chance of suffering from other attacks.

1. Have any medication in close proximity

Start treatment immediately with over-the-counter Ibuprofen (Motrin, Advil) or naproxen (Aleve) However, you should not take aspirin, as it could make the attack much worse. If you've experienced an attack before and your doctor has prescribed a medicine for relief to take in the event of another attack one, then take your prescribed medication in the manner your primary care physician or doctor physician has advised. If you're currently taking a medication that reduces the amount of uric acid in order to lower the risk of having attacks, continue taking the medication throughout your current attack.

2. Ice down

Applying an ice-pack to the joint that is hurting can help ease the pain and irritation. Wrap the pack (a bag of squashed, frozen peas or ice work) in dish cloth and place it on the joint for 20-30 minutes, stretching a several times a day.

3. Contact your doctor

Let your primary care physician or doctor physician about the problem right away. They could give you a second prescription or send you to the lab to conduct a joint fluid analysis (to confirm a diagnosis of gout) or injecting corticosteroid in order to begin slowing the process of reducing inflammation. The treatment you receive within the first 24 hours following the onset of an attack could reduce the duration and severity.

4. Take a large amount of liquids

Staying hydrated can help eliminate uric acid (the reason behind your joint discomfort) and prevent kidney stones. This is another issue that could be caused by elevated levels of uric acids. Drink 8 or 16 cups fluids every day, and make sure that at least half comprise water.

5. Avoid drinking alcohol

Despite your feelings that could be tempted to take drinks to ease the tension in the event of pain, it's vital to stay clear of spirits, specifically beer, which is a source of large amounts of purines. Uric acid is produced by the body in the process of processing purines. In addition, alcohol hinders the elimination of uric acids out of the body.

6. Find a walking stick

Utilizing a walking stick in Gout attacks that are intense could aid in keeping weight off of the joint that is causing pain.

7. Releasing your feet if they are affected

Lifting your feet by using cushions, so they're more elevated than the chest can help lessen swelling.

8. Make sure you are able to control your sheets

In fact, even the weight of your sheets can be a strain on the toe, which is irritated and gouty. Make sure the sheets are secured along the sides, so that its bottom is at the level of your calf and leaves your toe in pain free.

9. Create gout-friendly socks

Cut the portion of the socks that are designed for the large toe from any low-cost pair of socks that you have, or cut off a small portion of the socks designed for the entire toe section.

10. Relax

Try to loosen the tension whenever you are able; stress may cause gout to worsen. Go to a motion movie or converse with a friend or read a book, or listen to music

11. Change the menu

Stop eating foods that have high levels of purine like red meat, shellfish sweetbreads, sauces, and sweetbreads.

The Most Effective Ways To Avoid Gout Attacks

To prevent painful repeats of gouty joint pain check your uric level and follow the proper doses of medication.

Gout is a painful joint disorder that affects 3.4 millions of American men. It was once referred to by the name of "sickness of lords" as because of its association with the excessive blue-blooded use of mead and lamb but the reason behind it is more or less rational: Gout-related attacks occur when uric acid, which is a chemical produced in the body, increases to an unnatural level and starts to form crystals within the joint affected. This can cause irritation and extreme pain, sometimes accompanied by muscular aches, fever and other signs of flu.

In 2012 in 2012, the American College of Rheumatology (ACR) issued its first ever directive to prevent and treat Gout. If you're at risk of suffering from gout, one best way to escape the gout-related ailment is to keep the level of uric acids below 6.0 milligrams/deciliter (mg/dL) in accordance with the guidelines that is issued by the College of Rheumatology. If you're suffering from a lot of episodes of gout, it's important to be aware of your number.

Tips to help prevent Gout

Everyone will admit that gout prevention is crucial. Here are some helpful tips to help keep gout at bay.

1. Get your diet in order

It is well-established that gout can have a thing or two in common with your diet and it is logical to take steps to reduce it. To help you Here are some food items you ought to avoid as much as you can in order to avoid gout:

Corn syrup with high-fructose content

Meat from organs

- Excess liquor

Here are a few food items that you should consume in small quantities:

Large portions or portions of fish and meat.

- Regular sweet fruit juices

Sugar, pastries and salt

Here are some foods that you should eat more of:

Low-fat or nonfat dairy products

- Vegetables

In the ideal scenario, all you need to do is wipe out all triggers from your diet, as the diet is often associated by gout flare-ups and attacks. Refraining from triggers and adhering the proper diet that is suitable for gout is an effective remedy on its own.

Research has shown that red fish, meat as well as sugar and liquor are the most likely causes, it makes sense to avoid them , and stick to low-sugar organic food items such as vegetables, whole grains fruit, nuts and dairy that have been proven as healthier.

2. Changes in lifestyle

When there is something going on with our bodies it's a sign that we're doing something wrong , and there are some lifestyle changes that we must take for our own benefit. This is especially true for gout as most of the reasons can be related to the way you conduct every day and also the lifestyle that you've absorbed. A few lifestyle changes that are necessary in order to prevent getting gout attacks are:

You can lose some weight if you're overweight.

Stop smoking

- Create an exercise routine

Drink water frequently

Consuming plenty of water is vital for kidney function. Maintaining the kidneys in good shape as they should be a good way to reduce the growth of crystals of uric acid and Gout attacks.

Make sure you stay hydrated and drink plenty of water. This can be beneficial for Gout. There is no evidence to suggest that it could replace gout medications but it could be useful.

Take a good amount of rest

Gout-related attacks can affect the ability to work and mobility. To prevent the onset of symptoms, you should unwind the muscles and loosen them when joints are affected by inflammation. Avoid exercising or putting on a lot of weight and using joints for too long and this can increase the severity and duration of the attack.

Chapter 5: Treatment Of Gout

The purpose in this section is to go beyond understanding how to manage your self during an attack of gout and how to to prevent attacks from happening again. In this chapter, we will dive deep into the treatment for Gout. Of course, there are certain aspects that could be repeated. But the goal isn't to be repeated and uninteresting. The goal is to put an emphasis on the most important aspects, such as the medications prescribed for the treatment of Gout.

Gout attacks are sudden and cause sharp pain usually in a particular and isolated joint. Big toes are the primary part of the body which is affected by the. The release of uric acid could trigger gout attacks.

Some people will generally produce an enormous amount of uric acid , without having an obvious reason. For others, the problem is a poor functioning kidney that isn't able to keep up with the amount of uric acids being released. The use of diuretics ("water tablets") for hypertension can also contribute to the increase in production of uric acid that may cause the onset of gout.

Certain foods may increase the chance of suffering from attacks of gout. These gouty food items contain purines, synthetic compounds that disperse within the body to create the uric acid. The most likely culprits are meat sauces, red meat along with fish and alcohol (particularly alcohol). Certain vegetables also increase levels of urinary acids. Some of them are beans, lentils as well as asparagus, mushrooms peas, cauliflower and spinach. Additionally, corn syrup that has high fructose content has been linked to gout.

But, only 10% of urine produced in the body comes from food. If the uric acid level is high changing your diet do not suffice to lower it to a normal level. It's not as efficient as people say.

However do not ignore the diet. Minimizing your beer intake may lessen gout attacks. In overweight individuals, losing the weight of a couple of pounds makes an impact. Evidence suggests that eating fruit regularly can reduce your risk of developing gout slightly, but how much it aids is not clear.

The Job Of Drugs In Gout Treatment

Certain indicators suggest the need for regular usage of drugs. The signs are repeated attacks (a couple of times per year) or extreme attacks that are difficult to manage, gout that has the background of kidney stones or gout that is affecting several joints. The latest ACR rule states that kidney disease is a sign of the need for medication to decrease the levels of uric acid.

The ACR also supports higher doses of uric acids reduction drugs to reduce levels to less than 6.0 mg/dL. Before, doctors recommended dosages of these medications which were excessively low to avoid the effect on kidney functions.

It's not the case that everyone with gout has to be taking a uric-acid reduction medicine. Certain groups of people, just having high levels of uric acid in your blood won't always cause the gout. In addition, a handful of people experience attacks in a variety of ways and are able to manage them by using a nonsteroidal painkiller (NSAID) in the event of flare-ups.

If you experience frequent attacks and the NSAIDs perform in a consistent manner, you might not require lifelong medical treatment.

Colchicine is the mainstay of treatment for gout for many years. The ACR recommends lower amounts of colchicine that are taken to ease gout attacks despite the fact that the drug can be used by only 33% of people within 24 hours. If someone is taking long-term uric-acid decrease medications using colchicine, it can lower the likelihood of suffering from gout attacks during the time it may take for the uric acid reduction medicine to show complete results.

Extremism: Overdoing it

Although a diet that is low in purine won't necessarily make a man with gout immune to the acrid symptoms from "the disease of kings," there are plenty of valid reasons to cut down on your consumption of meat, and to enjoy your beer and fish in smaller amounts.

Red meat-based diets are linked to cancer and coronary diseases. Drinking a lot of alcohol or mixed drinks won't cause an incredibly severe gout attack in the future. But it's not good for your heart and can lead to weight growth. There are no benefits to drinking more than a few drinks that are sweetened with high-fructose corn syrup.

Step-by-step directions for treating Gout Attacks home

If you suffer from gout you're aware of the warning symptoms that indicate that an attack is on the way. There's no way in order to stop the attack when it has begun, however, you can treat some or the signs at home.

Warn signs that you're likely to suffer from Gout attack

Many people suffering from Gout, also known as gouty arthritis, claim that the attack is triggered by an intense burning, tingling or itching sensations in the joint, which could last for one or two hours prior to the beginning of a flare-up. The joint might feel stiff or a little sore. Soon after signs of gout begin. If you experience frequent attacks, you'll become acquainted with the body's signal that indicates that attacks are about to commence.

Sometimes, people suffering from gout don't show any indications of a flare-up to occur. They might awake in the mid-night with a joint that is extremely painful.

When the flare-up is beginning there are a lot of people who suffer from swelling, redness, and severe pain generally within one joint. The most commonly recognized location for gout is the bottom of the large toe. It can also occur in a variety of joints, including the knee, elbow lower leg, wrist and even instep.

Home Care For A Gout Attack

If your primary doctor has diagnosed you with Gout and prescribed you medication to treat an attack, use the prescribed medication in the event that you discover you're experiencing one. In general, this is likely to be when you notice the first signs begin to appear.

Your doctor may recommend nonsteroidal anti-inflammatory drugs (NSAIDs) like meloxicam,indomethacin, sulindac or celecoxib or propose you make use of over-the-counter NSAIDs, such as naproxen or ibuprofen. Based on what your health history is, your doctor might recommend steroids or other treatments to reduce inflammation, such as colchicine (Colcrys).

In certain instances there is a possibility of using drugs such as colchicine for reasons of prevention. Your physician may have advised:

- Allopurinol (Aloprim, Lopurin, Zyloprim)

- Probenecid (Probalan)

- Rasburicase (Elitek)

- Lesinurad (Zurampic)

- Canakinumab (Ilaris)

- Pegloticase (Krystexxa)

If you are unable to take allopurinol, or isn't a viable option the doctor might suggest Febuxostat (Uloric). It is recommended to use it with caution, particularly due to the fact that it's been linked to an increase in the risk of dying from coronary illnesses and other causes.

If you're experiencing a flare-up, it does not mean that the medication isn't working. In the initial few months you are taking these medications, you could experience an attack while your body adjusts to the drug. Your physician may have prescribed you a medication to do in the event of an attack and.

If you've been taking a preventive Gout medication for time and are experiencing flares with no precedent for some period of time, consult your physician. They might talk to you regarding adjusting the dosage you're using or the medication itself.

The relief from discomfort is not a prescription

1. Utilize cold

If the pain isn't painful, try giving compresses or cold packs a shot applying it to the joint to reduce inflammation and ease the pain. Place ice into a small towel and then apply it to the joint for up to 20 minutes, a few times throughout the day. Do not allow ice to touch your feet or hands in case you suffer from nerve problems due to diabetes or other reasons.

2. Relax the joint

It's an excellent idea to lay it down until the pain subsides. There's a good chance that you don't have a need to move it in any way. If there's a method to accomplish this you can raise the joint onto the pillow or some other material.

3. Drink water

If your body isn't drinking enough fluids or is dehydrated, levels of uric acid rise significantly higher. Stay hydrated in order to maintain your levels.

4. Be aware of what you eat and drink.

Foods high in purines or substances, for instance, certain fish, organ meats such as liver, as well as greasy food items could cause the uric acid levels up in your blood more. Also, fructose-sweetened drinks and liquor , particularly beer.

What is the best time to seek assistance for flare-up of gout?

It's always a good idea to inform your doctor that you're suffering from an episode of. At times it's possible to visit your doctor for a check-up to determine if your treatment is working , or if symptoms aren't getting better. Consult your physician when:

1. This is the first time you've attacked

There are many different diseases, such as joint disorders, that exhibit the same signs of Gout attacks. In this case, it is important to consult your physician and make sure that it is a gout attack , and not a different condition.

2. You're suffering from a fever and chills

Gout attack symptoms can include mild fever, but the presence of a fever could be a sign of a illness.

3. The symptoms do not improve after 48 hours or stop for seven days after that.

If you don't improve in some way after a few days, talk to your physician. They might suggest a different treatment. Gout attacks that are frequent will go away by themselves in a short period of time regardless of treatment.

Use Of Natural Remedies For Gout Treatment

If you're looking to try the natural cures This section is designed ideal for you. It is crucial to keep in mind that although natural remedies are beneficial however, you should not test these remedies if you suffer from allergies. Also, they do not replace medications prescribed by your physician.

Cherry fruit or tart cherry fruit juice

According to a survey from the year 2016 surveyTrusted Source The cherriesregardless of whether they are sweet red, sour, dark concentrated, as raw or as a juice cherries are incredibly popular and could be beneficial home remedies for many.

The 2012 study and the one in the same year also recommended testing cherries in order to avoid attacks of gout.

The study recommends three servings of cherries in two days that was deemed to be to be the most effective.

-Magnesium

Magnesium is a mineral which must be included on your food list. There are some who believe that it is beneficial to treat gout because the deficiency of magnesium could increase the inflammation stress within the body. But no research has definitively proved this.

In all likelihood, a study published in 2015 by Trusted Source revealed that taking the right amount of magnesium can lead to lessening and more beneficial levels of uric acid, and in this way, possibly reducing the risk of gout. The study was conducted on men, however there were no women involved in the study.

Take a shot at magnesium supplements. However, make sure to read the descriptions on the supplements carefully. On the other hand take magnesium-rich food every all day. This can reduce the risk of gout or the likelihood of developing gout over the long term.

-Ginger

Ginger is a common ingredient in cooking and is an herb suggested for inflammatory instances. Its ability to treat Gout is widely reported.

One study discovered that ginger applied topically decreased pain that is associated as gout uric acid. Another study found that for those with high levels of uric acids (hyperuricemia) their blood uric levels were decreased due to ginger. It is true it was rodents and ginger was taken internally, rather than applied topically.

Make an ginger paste or compress with 1 tablespoon fresh ginger root in water. Place a washcloth into the mixture. Once the washcloth is cool then place it on the area in which you're experiencing discomfort at least every other throughout the day for 15 to 30 minutes. A skin reaction or irritation could be a possibility, therefore it's best to conduct an experiment on a small portion of your skin first.

Intake ginger for internal use by taking two tablespoons of the ginger root for 10 mins in water boiling. Consume 3 cups each day.

Interactions between ginger and the medicines you're taking are possible. Make sure your doctor is aware beforehand before taking many doses of ginger.

Warm water with lemon juice, turmeric and vinegar from apple juice.

The combination of lemon juice and turmeric along with apple juice vinegar is frequently advised, especially to treat gout. Together, they are wonderful drinks and a natural solution.

There is no solid evidence to support apple juice vinegar as a remedy for Gout. However, studies suggest that it can help strengthen kidneys. However, research into the potential of turmeric and lemon juice to reduce blood uric acids levels is encouraging.

Mix the juice of one half lemon squeezed in warm water. Mix it in with 2 teaspoons of turmeric and 1 teaspoon vinegar from apple juice. Mix it until you are able to enjoy the flavor. Drink a few times daily.

Celery or celery seeds

Celery is a common food item used to treat urinary problems. To treat gout, concentrate and seeds of this vegetable have proven to be popular home remedies.

The trial use of the drug is widely reported. But, research based on logic is not sufficient. However, there is a suggestion that celery could reduce inflammation.

A sufficient amount of celery for treating Gout aren't mentioned. You can try eating celery every day especially raw celery sticks, juices , juice or seeds.

If you're buying an extract or supplement be sure to review the label carefully, and follow the instructions carefully.

-Nettle tea

Stinging bramble, also known as the nettle (Urtica dioica) is a common remedy to gout that can help reduce discomfort and inflammation.

The usage of customary methods is often alluded to in research studies. There isn't a single study concluding that it is effective. One study showed that it's great for kidneys. The subjects were male hares. the damage to kidneys was caused by the administration of an antibiotic known as Gentamicin.

In order to make the tea prepare the tea, boil a cup water. Soak one to two tablespoons dried nettle in a glass of water. Drink 3 cups per day.

-Dandelion

Dandelion tea concentrates, as well as supplements can be used to boost kidney and liver health.

They could lower the level of uric acids in people susceptible to damage to the kidneys as evidenced in two recent studies couple of years apart. But, these studies were conducted using rodents. Dandelion isn't an effective cure for Gout.

It is possible to use dandelion tea, concentrates, or as a supplement. Make sure you follow the label and follow the directions.

-Milk Thorn seeds

Milk thorn is a plant used to improve the health of your liver.

A recent study recommended that it could lower the level of uric acids in cases which can harm kidneys. A different report in 2013 confirms this suggestion. But, both tests were conducted on rodents.

Be sure to follow the dosage instructions for a milk-thorn supplement with caution or seek advice from your physician prior to making the decision to try it.

-Hibiscus

Hibiscus is a typical plant which can be consumed as a food item, drunk in tea, or utilized as a common home remedy.

In certain areas there is an alternative local treatment used to treat Gout. One study found that hibiscus could reduce the levels of uric acid. But, the study was carried out on rodents.

Use a tea, supplement or concentrate. Learn and follow the instructions when you are using it.

Topically hot or cold water or compress

Application

The application of cold or high-temperature, cold fluid to otherwise inflamed or troublesome joints can also prove beneficial.

The research and opinions on this topic are mixed. Injecting the joint, body part of the body, in cold water is often suggested and is thought to be the most effective. Ice packs can also help. Hot water soaks are generally only recommended when inflammation is less severe.

Alternating between cold and hot compresses or water applications can be extremely beneficial.

-Apples

Numerous natural wellbeing websites and blogs recommend apples as an integral part of diets to reduce gout. The reason is that apples are rich in malic acid that helps in bringing down the amount of uric acid.

There is no research to support this in the case of Gout. The fruit also contains fructose which could trigger hyperuricemia and which can trigger flare-ups of gout.

Consuming one apple a day can be beneficial to your overall well-being. It may be helpful in treating gout. But, only in the case that it does not add an excessive sugar consumption.

-Bananas

The fruit is believed to be helpful to treat Gout. They're rich in potassium, which aids organs and tissues of the body to function in a healthy way.

Bananas are also rich in sugars, like fructose. This can trigger gout. Many foods are rich in potassium and less sugar than bananas, such as dull greens, dull and boring avocados.

Take a banana a each day to gain an advantage. The research has not yet proven any benefit from bananas to treat Gout.

-Epsom salts

Some people recommend an Epsom salt bath to prevent gout attacks.

The theory is it is believed that Epsom salts are high in magnesium, which could reduce the risk of gout. In any event, StudiesTrusted Source shows magnesium cannot be absorbed sufficiently by the skin to offer any benefits for medical purposes.

To test Epsom salts Mix between 1 and 2 cups into the bathing water you use. Apply it to your entire body or only on certain joints, in the event of any negative side effects that result from the general use of skin care.

Chapter 6: Best Diet For Gout

The notion that "you are what you eat" isn't too far-fetched. Your diet will affect many aspects of your life, regardless of whether you're in good health. This is why it's essential to eat healthier and more nutritious when you suffer from an illness.

This chapter focuses on the most effective diet for gout, and the foods to avoid and based on the findings of research.

How Does The Food You Eat Affect Gout?

If you suffer from gout, certain foods could cause an attack by increasing your uric levels.

Trigger food items are typically rich in purines, which is which is a chemical that is typically found in food items. Uric acid is the waste result of the body's digestion of purines that are derived from food you've eaten.

It's not a problem for those who are healthy, because they are able to efficiently eliminate excess uric acids from their body.

But, people suffering from gout cannot effectively eliminate excess uric acids out of their body.

Therefore, a diet high in purine can allow uric acid to accumulate and trigger an attack of gout.

The good news is that research has proven that limiting the intake of high-purine food and taking the correct medicines can prevent attacks of gout.

Gout-related foods that are known to trigger attacks are organ meats such as liver red meats, fish as well as liquor and beer. They are a moderate to high amount of purines.

In any event there's a one exception to this rule. Research has shown that high purine vegetables don't cause attacks of gout.

Additionally, it is interesting to note that fructose and sweetened drinks may increase the risk of Gout and gout attacks even though they're not rich in purine. They can, however, increase the level of uric acids by stimulating some cell types.

For instance, research that included more than 125,000 people discovered that people who consumed the most fructose had a 62% increased likelihood of having gout.

However, research has shown that foods that are low in fat such as dairy and soy products and vitamin C supplements could assist in the prevention of gout attacks through decreasing the levels of blood uric acids.

High-fat and full-fat dairy products don't seem to affect the level of uric acids.

In all of this there are two main factors to keep in mind at into consideration when you are taking your health to. The first is that food items can elevate or decrease your uric acid levels depending on the purine levels. In addition, fructose could raise the levels of uric acids even though it's not purine-rich.

What Foods Would It Be A Good Idea For You To Avoid?

If you're susceptible to sudden attacks of gout be sure to stay clear of the primary triggers with regard to fooditems containing high levels of purine food items.

They are food items that have more than 200 milligrams of purines per each 3.5 pounds (100 grams).

Also, you should be wary of foods that contain high levels of fructose and foods that are high in purines that contain between 150 and 200 mg of purines per 3.5 grams. They could cause gout attacks if you consume them regularly.

Below are some foods with high levels of purine moderately high-purine food sources and food sources with high fructose to steer clear of.

1. Organ meats of all kinds Include liver, brain, kidneys and sweetbreads.

2. Meats from game: A few include venison, pheasant and veal.

3. Fish Sardines, mackerel herring anchovies and trout Tuna, Haddock Herring, mackerel, trout anchovies, sardines haddock, and many more.

4. Other seafood options: Roe, crab, shrimp, scallop, and scallop.

5. Sugary drinks: Specifically, fruit juices as well as soft drinks that contain sugar.

6. Sugars added to the diet: High-fructose corn syrup, sweetened with agave and honey.

7. Brewer's yeast nutritional yeast, as well as other yeast supplements

Additionally, refined carbohydrates like cakes, white bread, and other sweets must be avoided. Despite the fact that they're low in purines and fructose, they're low in nutrients and could increase the levels of uric acid in your body.

In essence, if you suffer from gout, it is recommended to be cautious about things like game meats organ meats, seafood, and various other seafoods as well as sugary drinks, refined carbs along with added sugars and yeast.

What Foods Would It Be A Good Idea For You To Eat?

Although a diet that is gout-friendly excludes a lot of foods off the menu of food items that you are allowed to eat there's plenty of low-purine food items to enjoy.

Foods are considered to be low-purine when they contain less than 100mg of purines each 3.5 grams (100 grams).

Below are some foods with low levels of purine that are generally safe for people suffering from gout.

1. Fruits : All varieties of fruits are typically suitable for those suffering from Gout. They can even prevent attacks by lowering the levels of uric acid and reducing inflammation.

2. Vegetables: All veggies are delicious such as peas, eggplants mushrooms, extremely leafy, dark vegetables.

3. Legumes They are all fine which includes lentils, soybeans tofu, beans, and tofu.

4. Nuts Seeds and nuts are fine.

5. Full grains: Whole or full grains like brown rice, oats and barley are fine.

Dairy products: Every dairy is great, but low-fat dairy is especially beneficial.

5. Eggs.

6. Drinks: Tea, green tea tea and coffee.

7. Spices and herbs: All herbs and spices are safe.

8. Plant-based oils: including coconut oil, flax oil, oil from canola as well as olive oil.

The Foods You Can Eat With Some Restraint

In addition to organ meatsand game meats and some seafood, the majority of meats are able to be consumed with a certain amount of caution. It is recommended to limit your consumption to 4-8 pounds (115-170 grams) of these at a handful of times per week.

They have a small amount of purines. This is considered to be between 100 and 200 mg per 100 grams. So, eating lots of them could cause a gout attack. Here are a few.

1. Meats: Some examples include pork, chicken, mutton and beef.

2. Certain kinds of fish can be canned or fresh in general contain less purines than the majority of other fish.

The main point to remember is that the food items you need to avoid eating with gout are any food that is grown from the soil, as well as grains, dairy products with low fat eggs, and generally drinks. Reduce your intake of nonorganic seafood and meats like salmon to portions of 4 to 6 8 ounces (115-170 grams) at least once each week.

Other Lifestyle Changes You Can Make

In addition to your diet In addition, there are lifestyle adjustments that will allow you to reduce your risk of suffering from gout or attacks with gout.

1. Lose weight

If you suffer from gout being overweight can increase the risk of having Gout-related attacks .

This is due to the fact that weight gain can cause you to become more resistant to insulin, which can lead to the development of insulin resistance. In these situations it is impossible for the body to utilize insulin in a way that allows sugar to be eliminated from blood. Insulin resistance can also increase the levels of uric acid in the blood.

Research has shown that becoming better fit can decrease the resistance to insulin and reduce the level of uric acids.

This being said that you must stay clear from crash diets and fad diets -- which means trying to slim down and become weightless quickly by eating less than you ought to. Studies have shown that a rapid weight loss can result in an increase in likelihood of suffering from gout attacks.

2. Exercise More

Exercise routinely is a different method to combat the effects of gout. Exercise is not just about helping to keep the weight that is right for you, it can help keep the levels of uric acids in check.

A study in 228 men discovered that those who ran 5 miles (8 kilometers) each day had an 80% lower chance of suffering from gout. This is partly due to the fact that they were less overweight.

3. Remain Hydrated

Drinking enough water can reduce the chance of suffering from Gout attacks.

It is because that a healthy intake of water allows the body to flush out excess uric acid from bloodstream, flushing it away through the urine.

If you're an active person, it's vital to stay hydrated because of the fact that you can lose quite a bit of water by sweating.

4. Beware of drinking alcohol.

Liquor is the most frequent trigger for gout attacks.

It is believed that the body might concentrate more on removing alcohol rather than eliminating uric acids which allows uric acid to build up and lead to crystal formation.

A study involving 724 people discovered that drinking alcohol such as beer, wine or other forms of alcohol increased the chance of suffering from gout attacks. A drink of one to two drinks every per day increases the danger by 36% and drinking two to four drinks per day increased the risk by 51%.

5. Consider taking a Vitamin-C Supplement

Certain studies suggest Vitamin C-rich supplements could aid in preventing gout attacks by decreasing the levels of uric acid.

It is believed that vitamin C works by aiding the kidneys in the efficient eliminate uric acid from the body by urination.

A study however concluded that the use of nutrient C supplements didn't have an effect on the condition of gout.

The research into vitamin C supplements to treat Gout is still in the beginning, and it is necessary to conduct more research before a definitive conclusion are reached.

In the end, it's crucial to remember that being more active by exercising, keeping well-hydrated, limiting alcohol consumption and most likely supplementing with vitamin C could assist in preventing attacks of gout.

Recipe 1:   Green Bean Chowder

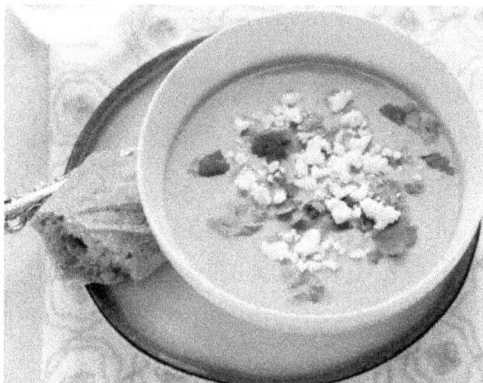

Beans are a valuable source of proteins and when used in a chowder you get to enjoy all these benefits in every bite.

Yield: 4

Preparation Time: 5 hours 30 minutes

Ingredient List:

- 1 cup green beans
- 14oz. can coconut milk
- 1 cup water
- 1 ½ tablespoon yellow curry paste
- 3 garlic cloves, minced
- ¼ cup orange juice

- ½ cup diced tomatoes
- ½ cup diced potatoes
- 1 tablespoon dried parsley
- ¼ teaspoon fresh thyme
- 1 tablespoon minced ginger
- 2 teaspoons sugar
- 1 teaspoon hot sauce
- Salt and pepper- to taste

Instructions:

1. Place green beans in the slow cooker.

2. Add the garlic, potatoes, ginger, sugar, hot sauce, and curry paste.

3. Pour the orange juice and water.

4. Cover and cook on high for 4-5 hours.

5. Add the remaining ingredients and cook for 20 minutes more.

6. Serve while still hot.

Recipe 2:   Zucchini Crab Cakes

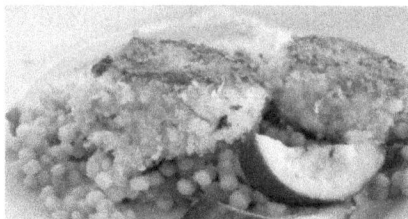

You don't need crab to enjoy delicious crab cakes.
Now you can enjoy the same amazing feeling
using zucchini.

Yield: 6

Preparation Time: 30 minutes

Ingredient List:

- zucchini (2 ½ cups, grated)
- egg (1, beaten)
- butter (2 tablespoons)
- Breadcrumbs (1 cup)
- onion (¼ cup, minced)
- Old Bay Seasoning (1 teaspoon)
- Flour (¼ cup)
- vegetable oil (½ cup, to be used for flying)

Instructions:

1. Combine all your ingredients, except oil and flour, in a large bowl and mix well.

2. Shape your mixture into 12 even patties, and dredge in flour.

3. Set a skillet over medium heat, add your oil and allow to get hot.

4. Fry your patties until perfectly golden on both sides.

5. Serve and enjoy.

Recipe 3:   Roasted Kabocha Squash

Kabocha squash is mildly sweet in flavor but

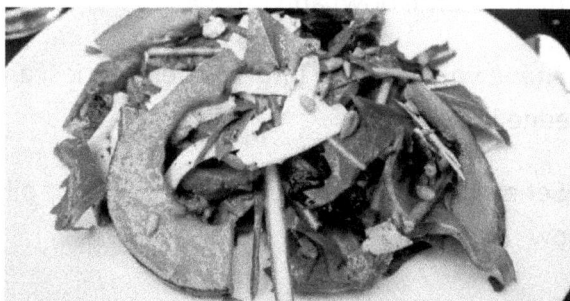

tends to go well with just about any protein as a side, or on its own as a snack.

Yield: 4

Preparation Time: 35 minutes

Ingredient List:

- Onion (1 small, chopped)
- Canola/Vegetable   Oil   (2 tablespoons)
- Rosemary (2 tablespoons, chopped)
- Thyme (1 teaspoon, chopped)
- Salt (¼ teaspoons)
- Pepper (1/8 teaspoons)

- Kabocha Squash (1 ½ lbs., skin on, washed and cut into even chunks)

Instructions:

1. Set your oven to preheat to 450 degrees F, and grease your baking sheet then set aside.

2. In a large bowl create a rub by mixing together your rosemary, salt, pepper, onion, thyme, and oil.

3. Throw in your squash and toss until well coated. Line a ¬layer of squash onto your baking sheet ensuring that none overlaps.

4. Bake until squash is tender and light brown in color.

5. Serve.

Recipe 4:   Braised Balsamic Chicken

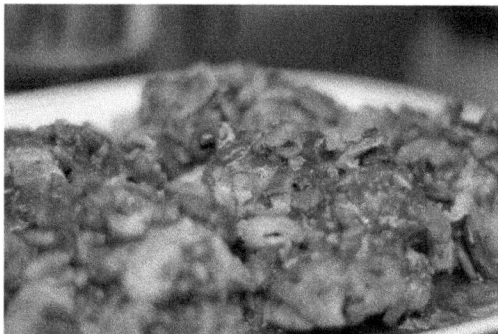

For a delicious low-fat, gout friendly dinner option be sure to try this Braised Balsamic Chicken.

Yield: 6

Preparation Time: 35 minutes

Ingredient List:

- chicken breast (6, skinless, halved)
- garlic salt (1 teaspoon)
- Black pepper (1 teaspoon)
- Olive oil (2 tablespoons)
- Onion (1, thinly sliced)
- tomatoes (14.5 ounces, diced)

- balsamic vinegar (½ cup)
- basil (1 teaspoon)
- oregano (1 teaspoon)
- Rosemary (1 teaspoon)
- thyme (½ teaspoons)

Instructions:

1. Use your garlic salt and pepper to lightly seasoned chicken breast and sets aside.

2. In a skillet, heat your olive oil over medium heat.

3. Next, add in your chicken then allow to cook until perfectly browned (about 4 minutes on each site).

4. Next, add onions and cook until fragrant (about another 4 minutes).

5. Add the remaining ingredients, and allows a similar until fully cooked (about another 15 minutes, the chicken should have an internal temp. of at least 165° F). Enjoy!

Recipe 5: Watermelon Juice

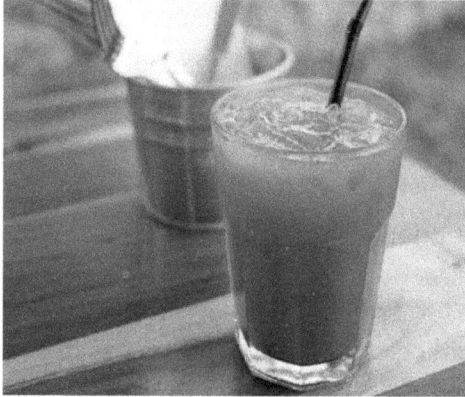

Watermelon is good for gout as it has a high water content, and water is great for flushing out your system.

Yield: 1

Preparation Time: 5 minutes

Ingredient List:

- 1 cup watermelon (seeds removed, and diced)
- 1 dash stevia powder
- 1 cup water

Instructions:

1. In a blender add all ingredients and blend well.

2. Serve and enjoy.

Recipe 6:   Slow – Cooker Vegetarian Chili

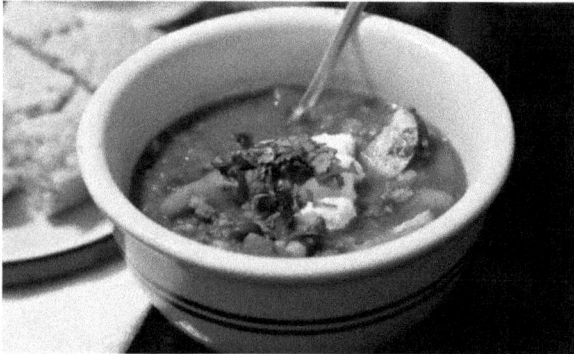

Now you can enjoy gout friendly twist off delicious gout friendly chili.

Yield: 8

Preparation Time: 2 hours 15 minutes

Ingredient List:

- Black bean soup (19 ounces)
- Kidney beans (15 ounces)
- Garbanzo beans (15 ounces)
- Baked beans (16 ounces, vegetarian)

- Tomatoes (14.5 ounces, canned, puréed)
- Corn (15 ounces)
- Onion (1, chopped)
- Bell Pepper (1, Green, chopped)
- Celery (2 stalks, chopped)
- Garlic (2 cloves, minced)
- Chili powder (1 tablespoon)
- Parsley (1 tablespoon, dried)
- Oregano (1 tablespoon, dried)
- Basil (1 tablespoon, dried)

Instructions:

1. Combine all your ingredients in a slow cooker, and allow to cook on high for about 2 hours. Enjoy!

Recipe 7: Turmeric & Pineapple Juice

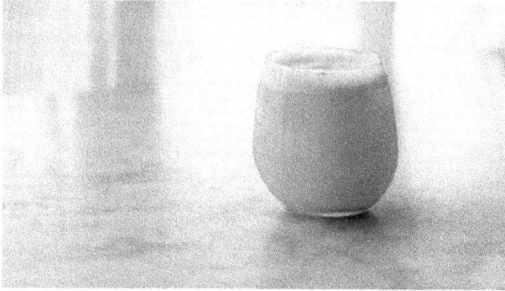

This mixture is rich in vitamin C and bromelain that are both great for reducing uric acid and relieving joint pain.

Yield: 1

Preparation Time: 5 minutes

Ingredient List:

- 1 cup pineapple (diced)
- 1 dash stevia powder
- 1 tablespoon turmeric
- 1 cup water

Instructions:

1. In a blender add all ingredients and blend well.

2. Serve and enjoy.

Recipe 8: Rosemary Watermelon Lemonade

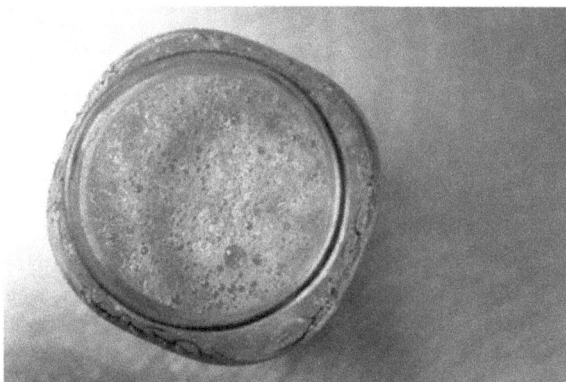

If you have trouble drinking water, this lemonade will be a good compromise.

Yield: 8

Preparation Time: 15 minutes + infusing time

Ingredient List:

- water (2 cups)
- sugar (¾ cup)
- Rosemary (1 sprig, leaves, chopped)
- lemon juice (2 cups)
- watermelon (12 cups, cubed)
- ice (8 cups)

Instructions:

1. In a medium saucepan, allow your water and sugar to come to a boil over high heat.

2. Once boiling, add your Rosemary, remove from heat, cover and allow to sit for at least an hour.

3. Strain your Rosemary syrup to remove rosemary leaves, then add all your ingredients to a blender.

4. Until smooth, strain, and serve over ice. Enjoy!

Recipe 9: Curried Fish

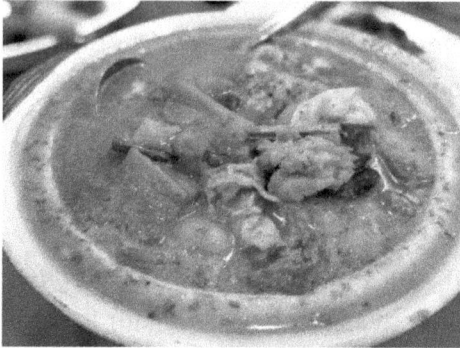

If you have never tried curried fish, then this may be the recipe for you.

Yield: 4

Preparation Time: 8 hours 10 minutes

Ingredient List:

- 1 teaspoon ground coriander seeds
- 2 tablespoons yellow curry paste
- 4 garlic cloves, minced
- 1 lb. cod, rinsed and dried then cubed
- ½ lb. green beans, cut into ½-inch pieces

- 1 cup finely chopped brown onion
- 4 small carrots, chopped
- 2 medium potatoes, cut into ½-inch slices
- ½ teaspoon cayenne pepper
- 1 ½ cup fish stock
- 1 cup coconut milk
- 1 teaspoon Fresh ground salt and pepper

Instructions:

1. Add your curry in a saucepan with oil over medium heat, and cook until fragrant (about a minute).

2. Add in your fish and allow to lightly brown in curry for about 2 minutes per side.

3. Combine all your remaining ingredients.

4. Cover and cook on medium for 20 minutes.

5. Season to taste, serve, and enjoy.

Recipe 10: Salsa Chicken Burritos

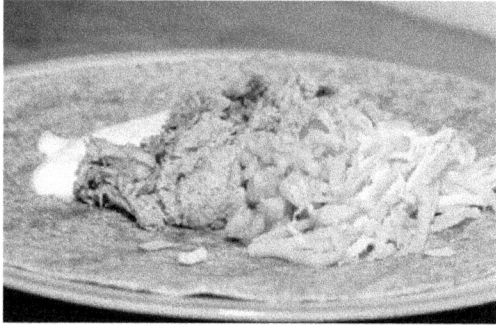

At a kick to your gout friendly menu by adding some salsa chicken burritos in the mix.

Yield: 4

Preparation Time: 35 minutes

Ingredient List:

- chicken breast (2 pieces, bone lessons skinless, halved)
- tomato sauce (4 ounces)
- salsa (¼ cup)
- taco seasoning (1.25 ounces)
- cumin (1 teaspoon, ground)
- garlic (2 cloves, minced)
- chili powder (1 teaspoon)

- Hot sauce (2 tablespoons)

Instructions:

1. Allow your chicken breasts to come to a boil with your tomato sauce over medium heat in a saucepan.

2. Once boiling, add any remaining ingredients and allow to simmer for at least 15 minutes.

3. Using a fork, pull your chicken into thin strings then return to the pot, cover and cook for at least 10 more minutes. Enjoy!

Recipe 11:   Cherry, Banana & Strawberry Smoothie

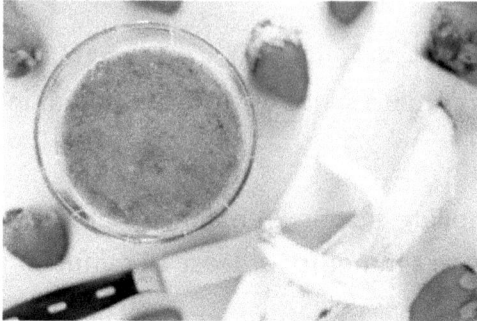

When you have gout it's important to stick to foods that provide you with the necessary anthocyanins to help relieve you of inflammation. Here is a recipe that will help you accomplish that.

Yield:2

Preparation Time: 15 minutes

Ingredient List:

- 2 cup cherries, frozen
- 1 ½ cup almond milk
- Banana (1, organic)
- Strawberries (1 cup, frozen)

Instructions:

1. In a blender add all ingredients and blend well.

2. Serve and enjoy.

Recipe 12:   Lemon Dill Salmon

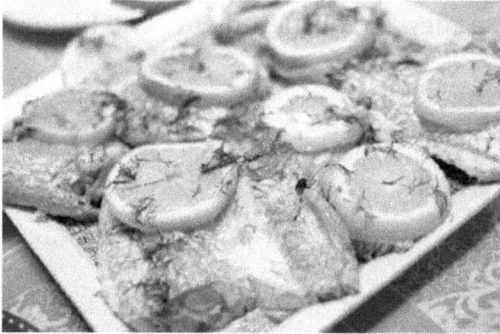

Selecting good gout friendly lunch can be difficult. Enjoy this delicious salmon dish knowing that it's not only gout friendly but delicious.

Yield: 4

Preparation Time: 35 minutes

Ingredient List:

- salmon (1 pound, fillets)
- butter (¼ cup, melted)
- dill weed (1 tablespoon)
- Garlic powder (¼ teaspoons)
- Sea salt (1 teaspoon)
- Black pepper (1 teaspoon)

Instructions:

1. Set your oven to preheat to 350° F and prepare a baking dish by lightly greasing.

2. Adding the salmon into the prepared baking this and drizzle your remaining ingredients on top.

3. Set to bake until salmon is fully cooked (about 25 minutes). Enjoy!

Recipe 13:   Brown Stewed Chicken

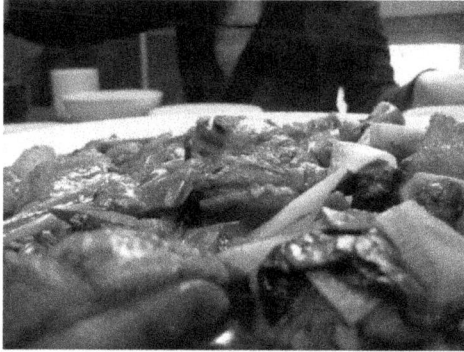

If soul-warming food is your cup of tea, then you need to try out this recipe.

Yield: 6

Preparation Time: 4 hours 15 minutes

Ingredient List:

- 3lbs chicken, sectioned
- 1 tablespoon Worcestershire sauce
- 14oz. can coconut milk
- ½ cup chicken stock
- 2 tablespoons fish sauce
- 2 tablespoons brown sugar
- 2 teaspoons browning

- 1 tablespoon lemon juice
- 2 limes, juiced and zested
- 1 tablespoon olive oil
- ½ teaspoon Salt
- ¼ teaspoon Pepper

Instructions:

1. Heat the oil in a dutch oven over medium-high heat. Season the chicken and cook in the oil until browned on all sides.

2. Add the Worcestershire sauce, brown sugar, and lemon juice. Cook until the sugar is melted.

3. Next, add in your remaining ingredients, cover and cook on high for 30 – 45 minutes.

Recipe 14:   Potato And Vegetable Frittata

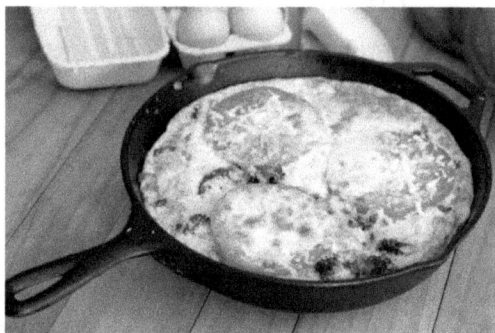

Here we have a delicious breakfast option for your gout friendly menu.

Yield: 2

Preparation Time: 25 minutes

Ingredient List:

- olive oil (1 teaspoon)
- Onion (½ cup, chopped)
- garlic (1 clove, minced)
- Bell Pepper (½ cup, diced, green)
- zucchini (1, cut into ¼ inch matchsticks)
- potatoes (2 cups, cooked, diced)

- tomato (1 cup, chopped)
- olives (2 tablespoons, Black)
- eggs (4, large)
- salt (1 teaspoon)
- black pepper (1 teaspoon)
- Oregano (¼ teaspoons)
- Cayenne pepper (¼ teaspoons)
- Cherry tomato (½, small, sliced)
- mozzarella (¼ cup, shredded)
- Parmesan cheese (¼ cup, grated)

Instructions:

1. Set your boiler to preheat to high.

2. Sauté your bell pepper, garlic, and onion with oil in an ovenproof skillet until tender.

3. Add your potatoes, and stir to combine.

4. Next, add your zucchini, tomatoes, and olives, and continue to stir until potatoes have become tender.

5. In a separate bowl, combine your egg and seasoning (cayenne pepper, black pepper, salt, and oregano) and whisk to combine.

6. Pour your eggs over your vegetable mixture in your skillet, arrange or cherry tomatoes on top of the eggs, top with cheeses, and allow to cook until eggs are almost set.

7. Place your skillet under your boiler until eggs have been fully set, and cheeses form a nice golden-brown crust. Serve and enjoy!

Recipe 15: Creamy Peanut Soup

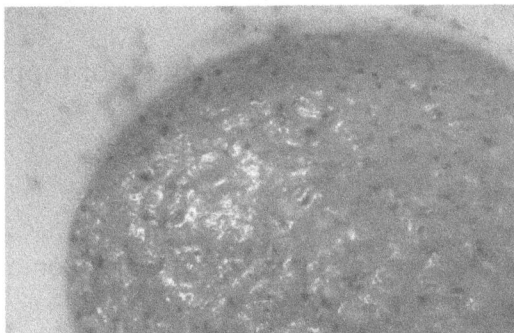

This bowl of soup will wow you!

Yield: 8

Preparation Time: 4 hours 10 minutes

Ingredient List:

- 4lb. skinless and boneless chicken breasts
- 2 tablespoons lime juice
- 4 cups chicken broth
- 4 tablespoon honey
- 1 cup peanut butter, preferably chunky
- 2 green bell peppers sliced

- 2 brown onions, diced
- 2 red bell peppers, sliced
- ½ cup soy sauce
- ½ cup crushed peanuts, for topping

Instructions:

1. Place the sliced bell peppers and diced onion in the bottom of slow cooker.

2. In a medium bowl, whisk the peanut butter, soy sauce, lime juice, honey, and chicken broth.

3. Cook on high for 30 minutes then transfer your soup to either a blender or food processor and pulse until smooth.

4. Sprinkle with peanuts, serve, and enjoy.

Recipe 16:   Honey Mustard Chicken

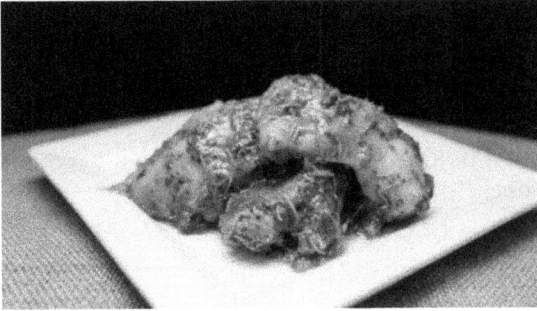

Here is a delicious gout friendly recipe that the whole family can enjoy.

Yield: 6

Preparation Time: 1 hour

Ingredient List:

- chicken breasts (6 pieces, boneless and skinless)
- salt (½ teaspoon)
- Black pepper (½ teaspoon)
- Honey (½ cup)
- mustard (½ cup, Dijon)
- basil (1 teaspoon)
- Paprika (1 teaspoon)

- Parsley (½ teaspoon, Dried)

Instructions:

1. Set your oven to preheat to 350° F, and prepare a baking dish by lightly greasing.

2. Season your chicken breasts by sprinkling with your salt and pepper.

3. Combine your remaining ingredients in a small bowl and mix well.

4. Brush a half of this mixture over chicken, and placed to bake for 30 minutes.

5. Turn the chicken pieces over, brush with your remaining honey mustard glaze, and allow to cook for another 15 minutes. Remove from heat and serve.

Recipe 17:   Lentil Soup

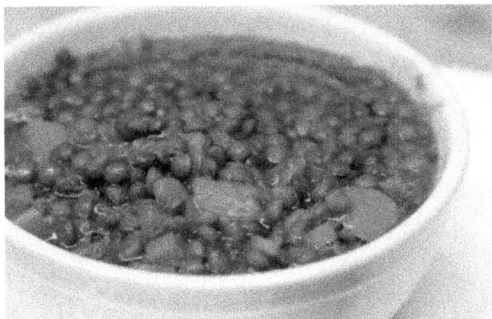

Enjoy this warm bowl of soup on a cold winter day.

Yield: 4

Preparation Time: 1 hour

Ingredient List:

- 1 cup brown lentils
- 4 cups vegetable broth
- ½ bay leaf
- ¼ teaspoon ground coriander seeds
- ½ tablespoon olive oil
- ½ teaspoon Salt
- ¼ teaspoon Pepper

Instructions:

1. Rinse the lentils under cold water and remove any black ones.

2. Place the rinsed lentils into a rice cooker.

3. Add the remaining ingredients and give it a good stir.

4. Cover and cook for 60 minutes.

5. Season to taste and serve while still hot.

Recipe 18:   Vanilla Fruit Salad

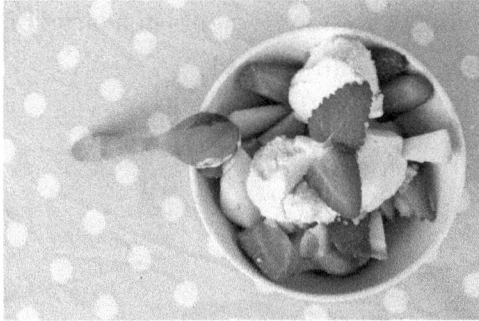

If you like sweet breakfast dishes, then this is a must try. This dish is filled with nutrients and antioxidants to help ease gout pain.

Yield: 6

Preparation Time: 15 minutes

Ingredient List:

- Apples (2 cups, diced)
- banana (1 cup, sliced)
- strawberries (1 cup, sliced, fresh)
- walnuts (1 cup, chopped)
- yogurt (1 cup, vanilla)
- cinnamon (¾ teaspoons, Ground)

Instructions:

1. Combine all your ingredients in a large bowl, stir gently. Serve and enjoy!

Recipe 19:   Spicy Pan-Fried Chicken

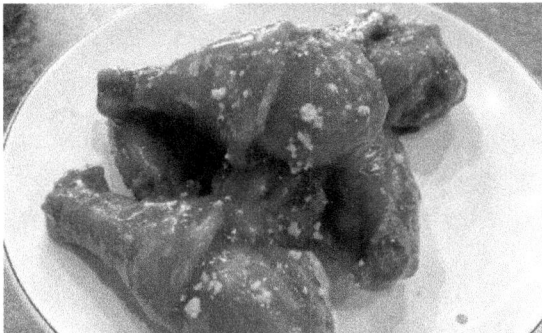

If you like spice then this is a tasty gout friendly recipe that will please your palate.

Serve: 3

Preparation Time: 30 minutes

Ingredient List:

- Chopped onion: ¼ cup
- Soy sauce: 5 tablespoons
- Minced garlic: 2 tablespoons
- Brown sugar: 2 ½ tablespoons
- Sesame oil: 2 tablespoons
- Sesame seeds: 1 tablespoon
- Cayenne: ½ tsp

- Salt and pepper
- Boneless chicken breasts, strips: 1 lb.

Instructions:

1. Take a bowl and mix all ingredients except chicken.

2. Put chicken in mixture and coat well.

3. Take a skillet and transfer mixture with chicken into it.

4. Cook on a medium heat for 20 minutes.

5. Serve, and enjoy.

Recipe 20: Slow Cooker Chicken Stew

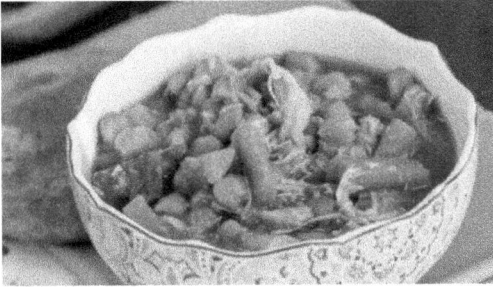

Consuming too much red meat is taboo for gout patients. This doesn't mean, however, that you can't enjoy a delicious stew.

Yield: 6

Preparation Time: 4 hours

Ingredient List:

- chicken thigh (2 lbs., cut into small pieces)
- flour (¼ cup, all-purpose)
- salt (½ teaspoons)
- Black pepper (½ teaspoons)
- Garlic (1 clove, minced)
- bay leaf (1)

- paprika (1 teaspoon)
- Worcestershire sauce (1 teaspoon)
- Onion (1, chopped)
- beef broth (1 ½ cups)
- potatoes (3, diced)
- carrots (4, sliced)
- celery (1 stalk, chopped)

Instructions:

1. Combine all your ingredients in a slow cooker, cover, and allow to cook on high for about 4 hours. Serve and enjoy!

Recipe 21:   Hoisin Chicken Filled
Lettuce Wraps

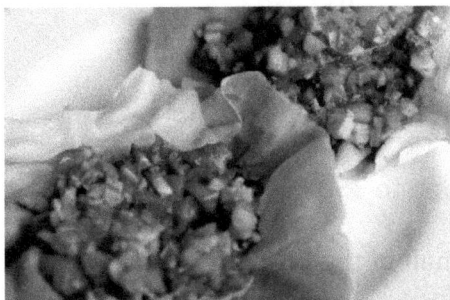

These wraps are typically a popular item in bars, and now you can enjoy them from your kitchen.

Yield: 4

Preparation Time: 25 minutes

Ingredient List:

- Chicken breasts (12 oz., sliced)
- Olive oil (2 teaspoons)
- Onion (1, chopped)
- Black pepper (¼ teaspoon)
- Butter Lettuce (12 leaves, washed and separated)
- Garlic (2 cloves, minced)
- Ginger Powder (½ teaspoon)

- Hoisin sauce (3 tablespoons)
- Sesame Seeds (1/8 cup, black, and white)

Instructions:

1. Set oven to 350°F.

2. Heat half of the oil in a skillet and add onion, and garlic then cook for about 3 minutes.

3. Add your chicken, and toss to combine. Add in your hoisin sauce, stir to combine, and place in oven to cook until done (about 10 minutes).

4. Spoon chicken mixture into butter lettuce leaves.

5. Serve, and enjoy.

Recipe 22:   Cherry Smoothie

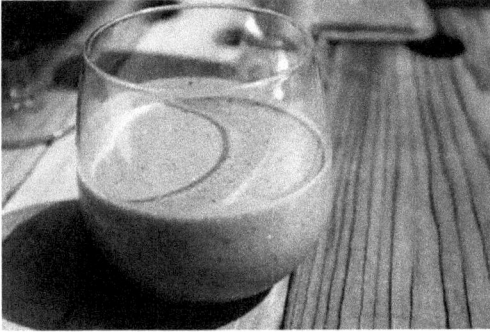

Cherries are known to help decrease inflammation levels in the body making it great for gout patients.

Yield:2

Preparation Time: 15 minutes

Ingredient List:

- 2 cup cherries, frozen
- 1 cup almond milk
- ½ cup coconut milk
- Few ice chunks (about 6)

Instructions:

1. In a blender add all ingredients and blend well.

2. Serve and enjoy.

Recipe 23:   Sweet & Spicy Chicken Wings

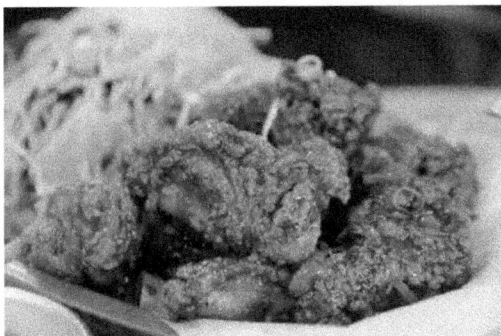

Chicken wings are thankfully fair game, even with gout.

Servings: 4

Preparation Time: 1 hour 30 minutes

Ingredient List:

- Chicken Wings (3 lbs.)
- Extra Virgin Coconut Oil (2 tablespoons)
- Garlic (4 cloves, chopped)
- Ginger (1 tablespoon, chopped)
- Siracha Sauce (3 tablespoons)
- Coconut Aminos (½ cup)

- Sherry (2 tablespoons)
- Honey (2 tablespoons)
- Apple Cider Vinegar (2 tablespoons)
- Fish Sauce (1 tablespoon)
- Peanut Oil (2 tablespoons)
- Salt (2 teaspoons)
- Black Pepper (1 teaspoon)
- Cajun spice (2 teaspoons)

Instructions:

1. Put wings into a large bowl, drain or pat to dry. Season well with salt, Cajun spice, and pepper, then set aside

2. In a small saucepan heat oil then add garlic, and ginger. Add all your remaining, and stir to create a sweet and spicy wing sauce. Remove from flame and add sesame oil.

3. Bake wings at 375 °until they are done.

4. Pour sauce mixture over wings and toss to coat.

5. Serve and enjoy!

Recipe 24:   Mushroom & Chicken Stuffed Bell Peppers

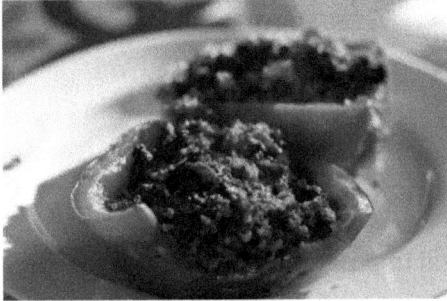

Here's a delicious dinner option that is fit for the whole family.

Yield: 4

Preparation Time: 35 minutes

Ingredient List:

- 1 cup Portobello mushrooms, chopped
- 2 red bell peppers, make a cut from stem
- 2 yellow bell peppers, make a cut from stem
- 1 cup chicken mince

- ½ cup tomato puree
- ¼ teaspoon garlic paste
- ½ teaspoon black pepper
- ¼ teaspoon salt
- 2 tablespoons olive oil

Instructions:

1. Heat oil in a pan and add garlic, fry for 1 minute.

2. Add chicken mince and mushrooms, then stir well.

3. When chicken mince becomes golden brown add tomato puree and fry again for 5-10 minutes.

4. Season with salt and pepper.

5. Preheat oven to 355 degrees.

6. Fill bell peppers with fried mince and place into greased pan.

7. Bake for 10 minutes.

8. Serve and enjoy.

Recipe 25: Grilled Chicken & Green Bean Salad

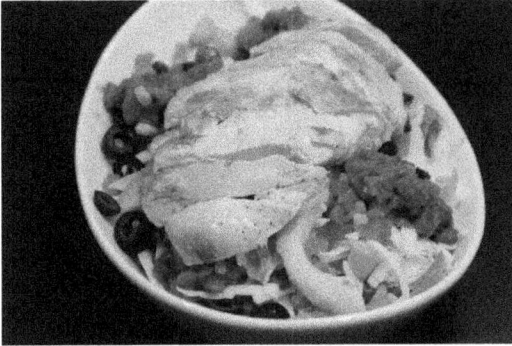

This salad is heaven to all chicken lovers.

Yield: 4

Preparation Time: 15 minutes

Ingredient List:

- Haricot Verts (¼ cup, blanched and chopped into halves)
- Basil (½ cup, chopped)
- Chicken (1 lbs., grilled, sliced)
- Olive Oil (4 tablespoons)
- Garlic (2 cloves, crushed)
- Salt (¾ tsp)

- Vinegar (2 tablespoons)
- Pepper (½ teaspoons)

Instructions:

1. In a small bowl, create a dressing by whipping together your vinegar, olive oil, garlic, salt, and pepper.

2. In another bowl add your remaining ingredients then pour the dressing over it.

3. Toss until evenly coated.

4. Serve and enjoy!

Recipe 26:   Chicken Mince Salad

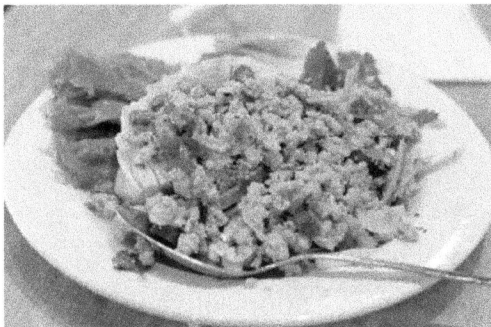

This delicious salad will keep you fuller longer.

Serves 4

Preparation Time: 35 minutes

Ingredient List:

- 1 oz. minced chicken
- Mint (1/3 cup)
- 1 onion, chopped
- 1 head baby cos lettuce, washed and separated
- 1 cup tomato puree
- ¼ teaspoon garlic paste
- ½ teaspoon chili powder

- ¼ teaspoon turmeric powder
- 1 bunch fresh coriander, chopped
- 1 lemon
- 2 green chilies
- ½ teaspoon cumin powder
- ½ teaspoon cinnamon powder
- 2 cups chicken broth
- ¼ teaspoon salt
- 2 tablespoons olive oil

Instructions:

1. Heat oil in a pan and add onion, fry for 2 minutes.

2. Add chicken mince with garlic and fry well until nicely golden.

3. Add tomato puree and fry again for 5-10 minutes.

4. Add salt, chili powder, turmeric powder. Stir.

5. Add remaining ingredients, and cover with lid. Leave to cook on low heat for 15 minutes.

6. Transfer lettuce onto a serving dish and top chicken mince.

7. Squeeze lemon juice.

8. Serve and enjoy.

Recipe 27:   Garlic Mashed Red Potato

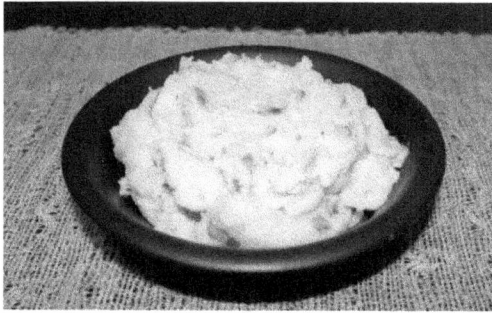

Enjoy this hearty mash as a delicious side dish.

Yield: 4

Preparation Time: 30 minutes

Ingredient List:

- Red Potatoes (2 cups, diced, cooked)
- Garlic (8 cloves, crushed)
- Olive Oil (6 tablespoons)
- Butter (½ cup, unsalted)
- Salt (1 teaspoon)
- Pepper (¾ teaspoon)
- Green Onions (1 stalk, diced)
- Radishes (4, medium, sliced)
- Carrot (1 medium, diced)

- Sweet Pepper (1 medium, diced)

Instructions:

1. In a large bowl, thoroughly combine all your ingredients until fully incorporated.

2. Mash with a potato masher, serve and enjoy.

Recipe 28:   Roasted Carrot & Bell Pepper Soup

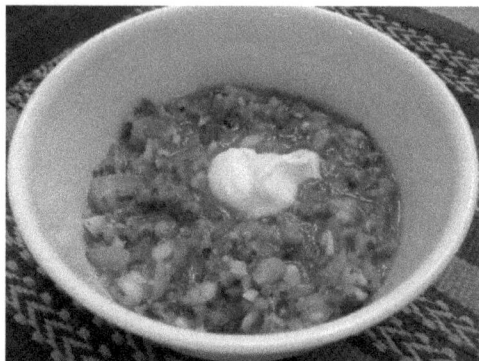

Enjoy this bowl of low cholesterol vegetable soup.

Yield: 5

Preparation Time: 35 minutes

Ingredient List:

- Extra Virgin Olive Oil (2 teaspoons)
- Shallots (½ cup, chopped)
- Bell Pepper (3 cups, roasted, peeled, cubed)
- Carrots (1½ cup, peeled, roasted, chopped)
- Ginger (1 tablespoon, grated)

- Chicken broth (3 cups, fat-free)
- Salt (¼ teaspoons)

Instructions:

1. Place a saucepan with your oil on medium heat until it just begins to smoke.

2. Add your shallots to the pot and sauté until it becomes tender (should take approximately 2 – 3 min).

3. Add the shallots all your prepped vegetables then allow to cook for another 2 minutes.

4. Pour in your broth and allow it to come to a boil. Once boiling, place the lid on the pot and reduce the heat to low.

5. Allow this mixture to simmer until your vegetables are all tender. Once tender, add salt and pour your soup into a food processor.

6. Pulse until creamy and smooth. Serve and Enjoy.

Recipe 29:   Sunomono Salad

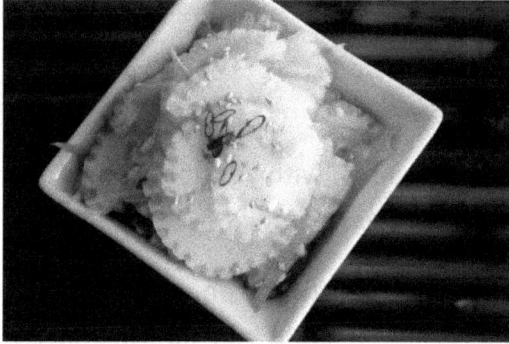

This salad is simple to make and creates the perfect snack.

Yield: 4 – 6

Preparation Time: 10 minutes

Ingredient List:

- Cucumber (1 English, thinly sliced)
- Rice Vinegar (½ cup)
- Sugar (2 tablespoons)
- Coriander Seeds (2 teaspoons, toasted)
- Salt (½ teaspoons)
- Red Pepper Flakes (¼ teaspoons)

Instructions:

1. In a medium-sized serving bowl thorough mix all the ingredients together until well incorporated minutes. Serve and enjoy!

Recipe 30:   Sweet & Nutty Fruit Salad

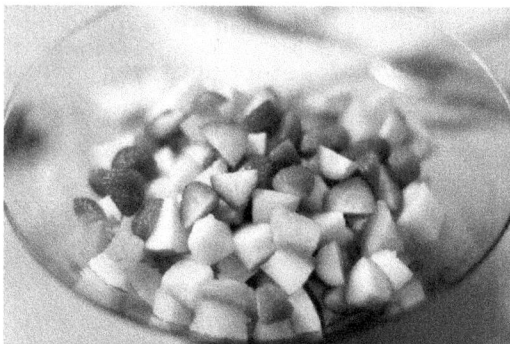

Here is a salad that even the kids will love.

Yield: 4

Preparation Time: 5 min

Ingredient List:

- Mayonnaise (2 tablespoons, low-fat)
- Lemon Juice (1 tablespoon)
- Apples (2 Granny Smith, small, cubed)
- Grapes (1 cup, red, halves)
- Cherries (1/3 cup, dried)
- Almonds (¼ cup, chopped)
- Grapes (¼ cup, sliced)

Instructions:

1. Create a dressing in a medium bowl by whipping the lemon juice and mayonnaise until fully combined.

2. Add your fruits, and almonds to the dressing and mix until fully coated.

3. Serve, and enjoy.

Chapter 7: What Is Gout?

Gout is an inflammatory type of arthritis that more commonly affects men. Gout causes sudden and severe joint pain that usually starts in the big toe. But other joints and areas around the joints can be affected, such as the ankle, knee and foot. It's the most common type of inflammatory arthritis. Men are three times more likely than women to develop gout. It tends to affect men after age 40 and women after menopause. Gout symptoms can be confused with another type of arthritis called calcium pyrophosphate deposition (CPPD). However, the crystals that irritate the joint in this condition are calcium phosphate crystals, not uric acid.

A medical history, physical examination and blood tests are used to diagnose gout. The doctor needs to know:

• How severe the pain is.

• How quickly it started.

• How long it has been happening.

• Which joints are affected.

The doctor will need to rule out other reasons for the joint pain and inflammation such as an infection, injury or other type of arthritis. The doctor may also take an X-ray, do an ultrasound or order a magnetic resonance imaging scan (MRI) to examine soft tissue and bone. The doctor might also remove fluid from the painful joint and examine it under a microscope for uric acid crystals or bacteria indicating an infection.

Treating An Acute Gout Attack

Here are the steps for getting the pain and swelling of gout attack under control as quickly as possible:

• Call your doctor and make an appointment.

• Ice and elevate the joint.

• Drink plenty of fluids (no alcohol or sweet sodas).

• Reduce stress, which can worsen the attack.

• Ask friends and family to help you with daily tasks to ease stress on joints.

Medications For Acute Gout Attack

Here are the medications that your doctor may prescribe at the first sign of an attack:

• Nonsteroidal anti-inflammatory drugs (NSAIDs) are frequently used to relieve the pain and swelling of an acute gout episode. They can shorten the attack, especially if taken in the first 24 hours.

• Corticosteroids: These drugs can be taken by mouth or injected into an inflamed joint to quickly relieve the pain and swelling of an acute attack. Corticosteroids usually start working within 24 hours after they are taken.

• Colchicine: This anti-inflammatory medicine works best if taken within the first 24 hours of a gout attack.

Reducing Uric Acid Levels

The doctor will wait until the acute attack ends before starting medications to reduce your uric acid levels. Sometimes, these drugs can cause an attack at first because uric acid levels drop and crystals in the joints shift. But sticking with the treatment plan is the best way to prevent future attacks. The doctor may prescribe a low, but regular dose of colchicine along with one of the medications below to prevent attacks.

Medications For Reducing Uric Acid Levels

The doctor will wait until the acute attack ends before starting medications to reduce your uric acid levels. Sometimes, these drugs can cause an attack at first because uric acid levels drop and crystals in the joints shift. But sticking with the treatment plan is the best way to prevent future attacks. The doctor may prescribe a low, but regular dose of colchicine along with one of the medications below to prevent attacks.

• Allopurinol (Zyloprim) reduces how much uric acid the body produces. It is often prescribed at a low daily dose at first, with which is increased slowly over time if uric acid levels remain high. This drug comes in pill form.

• Febuxostat (Uloric) reduces how much uric acid the body produces. Like allopurinol, it's started at a lower dose, which may be increased if uric acid levels remain high. This drug comes in pill form.

• Probenecid acts on the kidneys to help the body eliminate uric acid. The medication is taken twice daily and may be combined with febuxostat to boost effectiveness. This drug comes in pill form.

• Pegloticase (Krystexxa) is used when standard medications are unable to lower the uric acid level. It reduces uric acid quickly and to lower levels than other medications. The drug is administered every two weeks by intravenous (IV) infusion.

All drugs come with risks. To learn more about these drugs and their side effects, visit the drug guide.

Diet

Drink lots of water and avoid alcohol, beer, high-purine foods and sugary drinks to help reduce uric acid buildup.

Best Diet For Gout: What To Eat, What To Avoid

Gout is a type of arthritis, an inflammatory condition of the joints. It affects an estimated 8.3 million people in the US alone. People with gout experience sudden and severe attacks of pain, swelling and inflammation of the joints.

Fortunately, gout can be controlled with medications, a gout-friendly diet and lifestyle changes. Nearly half of gout cases affect the big toes, while other cases affect the fingers, wrists, knees and heels.

Gout symptoms or "attacks" occur when there is too much uric acid in the blood. Uric acid is a waste product made by the body when it digests certain foods.

When uric acid levels are high, crystals of it can accumulate in your joints. This process triggers swelling, inflammation and intense pain.

Gout attacks typically occur at night and last 3–10 days. Most people who have the condition experience these symptoms because their bodies can't remove the excess uric acid efficiently. This lets uric acid accumulate, crystallize and settle in the joints.

Others with gout make too much uric acid due to genetics or their diet.

How Does Food Affect Gout?

If you have gout, certain foods may trigger an attack by raising your uric acid levels. Trigger foods are commonly high in purines, a substance found naturally in foods. When you digest purines, your body makes uric acid as a waste product.

This is not a concern for healthy people, as they efficiently remove excess uric acid from the body. However, people with gout can't efficiently remove excess uric acid. Thus, a high-purine diet may let uric acid accumulate and cause a gout attack.

Fortunately, research shows that restricting high-purine foods and taking the appropriate medication can prevent gout attacks. Foods that commonly trigger gout attacks include organ meats, red meats, seafood, alcohol and beer.

They contain a moderate-to-high amount of purines.

However, there is one exception to this rule. Research shows that high-purine vegetables do not trigger gout attacks. And interestingly, fructose and sugar-sweetened beverages can increase the risk of gout and gout attacks, even though they're not purine-rich.

Instead, they may raise uric acid levels by accelerating several cellular processes. For instance, a study including over 125,000 participants found that people who consumed the most fructose had a 62% higher risk of developing gout.

On the other hand, research shows that low-fat dairy products, soy products and vitamin C supplements may help prevent gout attacks by reducing blood uric acid levels.

Full-fat and high-fat dairy products don't seem to affect uric acid levels.

What Foods Should You Avoid?

If you're susceptible to sudden gout attacks, avoid the main culprits' high-purine foods. These are foods that contain more than 200 mg of purines per 3.5 ounces (100 grams).

You should also avoid high-fructose foods, as well as moderately-high-purine foods, which contain 150–200 mg of purines per 3.5 ounces. These may trigger a gout attack.

Here are a few major high-purine foods, moderately-high-purine foods and high-fructose foods to avoid:

• All organ meats: These include liver, kidneys, sweetbreads and brain

• Game meats: Examples include pheasant, veal and venison

• Fish: Herring, trout, mackerel, tuna, sardines, anchovies, haddock and more

• Other seafood: Scallops, crab, shrimp and roe

• Sugary beverages: Especially fruit juices and sugary sodas

• Added sugars: Honey, agave nectar and high-fructose corn syrup

• Yeasts: Nutritional yeast, brewer's yeast and other yeast supplements

Additionally, refined carbs like white bread, cakes and cookies should be avoided. Although they are not high in purines or fructose, they are low in nutrients and may raise your uric acid levels.

What Foods Should You Eat?

Although a gout-friendly diet eliminates many foods, there are still plenty of low-purine foods you can enjoy.

Foods are considered low-purine when they have less than 100 mg of purines per 3.5 ounces (100 grams).

Here are some low-purine foods that are generally safe for people with gout:

• Fruits: All fruits are generally fine for gout. Cherries may even help prevent attacks by lowering uric acid levels and reducing inflammation.

• Vegetables: All vegetables are fine, including potatoes, peas, mushrooms, eggplants and dark green leafy vegetables.

• Legumes: All legumes are fine, including lentils, beans, soybeans and tofu.

• Nuts: All nuts and seeds.

• Whole grains: These include oats, brown rice and barley.

• Dairy products: All dairy is safe, but low-fat dairy appears to be especially beneficial.

• Eggs

• Beverages: Coffee, tea and green tea.

• Herbs and spices: All herbs and spices.

• Plant-based oils: Including canola, coconut, olive and flax oils.

Foods You Can Eat In Moderation

Aside from organ meats, game meats and certain fish, most meats can be consumed in moderation.

You should limit yourself to 4–6 ounces (115–170 grams) of these a few times per week.

They contain a moderate amount of purines, which is considered to be 100–200 mg per 100 grams. Thus, eating too much of them may trigger a gout attack.

• Meats: These include chicken, beef, pork and lamb.

• Other fish: Fresh or canned salmon generally contains lower levels of purines than most other fish.

A Gout-Friendly Menu For One Week

Eating a gout-friendly diet will help you relieve the pain and swelling, while preventing future attacks.

Here is a sample gout-friendly menu for one week.

Monday

• Breakfast: Oats with Greek yogurt and 1/4 cup (about 31 grams) berries.

• Lunch: Quinoa salad with boiled eggs and fresh veggies.

• Dinner: Whole wheat pasta with roasted chicken, spinach, bell peppers and low-fat feta cheese.

Tuesday

• Breakfast: Smoothie with 1/2 cup (74 grams) blueberries, 1/2 cup (15 grams) spinach, 1/4 cup (59 ml) Greek yogurt and 1/4 cup (59 ml) low-fat milk.

• Lunch: Whole grain sandwich with eggs and salad.

• Dinner: Stir-fried chicken and vegetables with brown rice.

Wednesday

• Breakfast: Overnight oats — 1/3 cup (27 grams) rolled oats, 1/4 cup (59 ml) Greek yogurt, 1/3 cup (79 ml) low-fat milk, 1 tbsp (14 grams) chia seeds, 1/4 cup (about 31 grams) berries and 1/4 tsp (1.2 ml) vanilla extract. Let sit overnight.

• Lunch: Chickpeas and fresh vegetables in a whole wheat wrap.

• Dinner: Herb-baked salmon with asparagus and cherry tomatoes.

Thursday

• Breakfast: Overnight chia seed pudding — 2 tbsp (28 grams) chia seeds, 1 cup (240 ml) Greek yogurt and 1/2 tsp (2.5 ml) vanilla extract with sliced fruits of your choice. Let sit in a bowl or mason jar overnight.

• Lunch: Leftover salmon with salad.

• Dinner: Quinoa, spinach, eggplant and feta salad.

Friday

• Breakfast: French toast with strawberries.

• Lunch: Whole grain sandwich with boiled eggs and salad.

• Dinner: Stir-fried tofu and vegetables with brown rice.

Saturday

• Breakfast: Mushroom and zucchini frittata.

• Lunch: Leftover stir-fried tofu and brown rice.

• Dinner: Homemade chicken burgers with a fresh salad.

Sunday

• Breakfast: Two-egg omelet with spinach and mushrooms.

• Lunch: Chickpeas and fresh vegetables in a whole wheat wrap.

• Dinner: Scrambled egg tacos — scrambled eggs with spinach and bell peppers on whole wheat tortillas.

Other Lifestyle Changes You Can Make

Aside from your diet, there are several lifestyle changes that can help you lower your risk of gout and gout attacks.

Lose Weight

If you have gout, carrying excess weight can increase your risk of gout attacks.

That's because excess weight can make you more resistant to insulin, leading to insulin resistance. In these cases, the body can't use insulin properly to remove sugar from the blood. Insulin resistance also promotes high uric acid levels.

Research shows that losing weight can help reduce insulin resistance and lower uric acid levels.

That said, avoid crash dieting that is, trying to lose weight very fast by eating very little. Research shows that rapid weight loss can increase the risk of gout attacks.

Exercise More

Regular exercise is another way to prevent gout attacks. Not only can exercise help you maintain a healthy weight, but it can also keep uric acid levels low.

One study in 228 men found that those who ran more than 5 miles (8 km) daily had a 50% lower risk of gout. This was also partly due to carrying less weight.

Stay Hydrated

Staying hydrated can help reduce the risk of gout attacks.

That's because adequate water intake helps the body remove excess uric acid from the blood, flushing it out in the urine.

If you exercise a lot, then it's even more important to stay hydrated, because you may lose a lot of water through sweat.

Limit Alcohol Intake

Alcohol is a common trigger for gout attacks. That's because the body may prioritize removing alcohol over removing uric acid, letting uric acid accumulate and form crystals.

One study including 724 people found that drinking wine, beer or liquor increased the risk of gout attacks. One to two beverages per day increased the risk by 36%, and two to four beverages per day increased it by 51%.

Try a Vitamin C Supplement

Research shows that vitamin C supplements may help prevent gout attacks by lowering uric acid levels. It seems that vitamin C does this by helping the kidneys remove more uric acid in the urine.

However, one study found that vitamin C supplements had no effect on gout. Research on vitamin C supplements for gout is new, so more studies are needed before strong conclusions can be made.

Gout Diet And Eating To Help Prevent Gout

Uric acid is a normal waste product in the blood that comes from the breakdown of certain foods. It's processed in the kidneys before being eliminated from the body in urine.

Excess Body Weight And Gout

Being overweight is associated with higher-than-normal uric acid levels. Since this is a major risk factor for gout, losing weight is often the goal of a gout diet.

Dieting And Weight Loss To Prevent Gout

Losing weight may help lower your uric acid levels and reduce your risk of future gout attacks. A 2017 review of studies in the Annals of the Rheumatic Diseases (1) suggested that a weight loss of about eight pounds or more led to long-term reductions in uric acid levels and gout attacks in overweight or obese people.

An Overview Of Dietary Approaches To Manage And Prevent Gout

The main principles of a gout diet are usually the same as those of any healthy, balanced diet. They include:

• If you're overweight, reduce the number of calories you consume.

• Choose unrefined carbohydrates like fruits, vegetables, and whole grains.

• Limit your intake of sugar-sweetened beverages and foods.

• Limit your intake of organ meats (such as kidney, liver, or sweetbreads).

• Cut back on saturated fats.

Dietary Causes Of Gout And Gouty Arthritis

Some people with gout find it helpful to eliminate specific high-purine foods from their diet. Certain high-purine foods may trigger gout attacks in some people. Most people with gout will still need medication even if they follow a diet for gout.

Dietary changes alone can lower your uric acid levels by up to 15 percent, according to the Institute for Quality and Efficiency in Health Care, an independent scientific institute that evaluates the benefits and harms of medical interventions.

Its not necessary to avoid all high-purine foods if you have gout. Studies have shown that purine-rich vegetables don't trigger gout. And certain high-purine foods can be a good source of lean protein to incorporate into your diet.

Purine-rich vegetarian foods to include in your diet are:

• Peas

• Beans

• Lentils

• Spinach

• Mushrooms

• Oats

• Cauliflower

• Broccoli

Foods To Avoid To Control Or Prevent Gout

The following foods may trigger gout attacks in some people:

• Red meat

• Organ meats

• Certain types of seafood (anchovies, sardines, herring, mackerel, scallops)

• Products containing high-fructose corn syrup

Drinks that can trigger gout include:

• Alcoholic beverages, especially beer, whiskey, gin, vodka, or rum

• Sugary drinks, including sodas, juices, energy drinks

• Coffee and other caffeinated beverages. While some studies show that caffeine can actually protect against gout pain, others find that sudden spikes in caffeine intake can trigger a gout attack.

Dietary Supplements For Gout Management And Prevention

Talk to your doctor about any supplements or vitamins you take or may want to take. Supplements and other remedies may interfere with medication.

Vitamin C supplements (up to 500 mg daily) are sometimes recommended for people with gout.

One study found that taking 500 mg of vitamin C per day had a mild uric-acid–lowering effect. Yet it's not clear whether vitamin C helps relieve gout symptoms.

A 2013 study in the journal Arthritis and Rheumatism showed that supplementing with 500 mg of vitamin C for eight weeks did not significantly lower uric acid levels in patients with gout.

Cherry Juice For Gout Management?

Cherries and cherry juice are a popular folk remedy for gout, but the scientific evidence to support their supposed benefits is still coming in. In 2005, the U.S. Food and Drug Administration sent warning letters to several cherry product manufacturers for overselling the health benefits of their products in advertisements.

Nonetheless, there's reason to believe that cherries may help fight gout. They contain chemical compounds called anthocyanins, which have been shown to help reduce inflammation.

Cherries may also have a beneficial effect on uric acid levels. One large study of people with recurrent gout found that eating cherries was associated with a lower risk of gout attacks, especially when cherry consumption was combined with taking a common uric acid–lowering drug.

Despite these findings, experts say that more research is needed before any definitive recommendations can be made about cherries or cherry juice for gout.

Chapter 8: Gout Recipes

Gout Recipes that include Salads, Dressings and other condiments.

When making your Gout diet work, you should include fresh vegetables whenever possible. Foods that are high in Vitamin C such as red cabbage, bell peppers,mandarins, oranges, potatoes.

When possible include pineapple as it is high in bromelain (friendly to the uric acid) , parsley, kale, green leaf vegetables, tuna, salmon , legumes, seeds, nuts, cherries, strawberries, blueberries , bananas, celery, tomatoes (small amounts), etc. But the most important thing is water. Lots of water per day, if possible up to 8 glasses, the more you drink the more your system will be flushed out.

These are important facts to consider for maintaining a healthy Gout diet.

Broccoli, Olives, & Egg Salad

Taco Salad:

4 chicken breast – boil, then shred with fork Olive Oil ,Cumin Chili Powder, 1 Can Rotel tomatoes with green chillies, 1 Large yellow onion – diced 1 Head Iceberg lettuce, 1 Can black olives, Shredded low fat cheddar cheese, low fat Sour Cream Guacamole (optional)

Homemade Salsa: 1 large can peeled tomatoes 1 small bunch cilantro 1 medium/large onion garlic salt to taste

How to Prepare:

In a large skillet, pour about 2 Tblsp olive oil and turn up to med/high heat. Sautee about 1⁄4 of the onions. Add the shredded chicken, cumin and chili powder and Rotel. Simmer for approximately 20 minutes, stirring occasionally. Meanwhile, shred lettuce and place in bowls. When Chicken mixture is done, place a heaping on top of the lettuce and cover with cheese, olives, low fat sour cream, the remaining onions. Combine salsa ingredients in blender. Add to salad. This will be used as your dressing. Enjoy.

Note; Try and use low fat ingredients for these Gout recipes.

Old Fashioned Cole Slaw

Serves: 8 Servings. Carbs Per Serving :6 grams carb 2 grams fiber (ECC=4)

Prep Time:<20 minutes Effort: Easy

Ingredients:

2/3 cup vinegar,

1/2 cup low fat whipping cream,

2 large eggs, lightly beaten,

1/4-1/2 cup Splenda Pinch of salt,

1 1/2 tablespoons butter cut into pieces,

1 (2-pound) head cabbage, shredded

How to Prepare:

Combine first 5 ingredients in a small, heavy saucepan; cook over low heat, stirring constantly with a wire whisk, 8 to 10 minutes or until thickened (mixture will appear curdled until it thickens).

Remove from heat. Add butter, stirring until it melts. Pour over cabbage; toss gently to coat. Cover and chill.

You can add 1/2 cup chopped walnuts and only raise the carb count by 1/2 gram. If you're on maintenance, 1/2 cup dried, chopped cranberries and the walnuts brings you in at a little under 10 grams.

Cranberry Salad

Serves: 8 Carbs Per Serving: 6.125g Effort: Easy

Ingredients:

1 can of crushed unsweetened pineapple – (9-oz.) juice,

1 package of sugar-free cherry gelatin – (.3-oz.)

1 tablespoon of lemon juice,

1/4 cup of artificial sweetener,

1 cup of fresh cranberries – chopped fine,

1 small orange – peeled, quartered and chopped small,

1 cup of celery – chopped 1/2 cup pecans – or other nuts, optional

How to Prepare:

Drain pineapple and save juice. Set pineapple aside for later use. Combine pineapple juice with water to equal 2 cups liuid. Prepare gelatin according to package label using juice-water mixture for the liquid. Once gelatin is dissolved, stir in lemon juice. Chill until partially set. In a separate bowl, combine the pineapple, sugar substitute, cranberries, orange, celery and nuts. Add this mixture to the partially set gelatin and stir until blended. Pour into large mold or individual molds. Chill until firm.

Do not use fresh or frozen pineapple in this recipe! It will not allow the gelatin to jell

Dijon Vinaigrette

Carbs Per Serving: 5g total

Effort: Easy

Ingredients:

3 tablespoons of red wine vinegar ,

2 tablespoons of water,

1 tablespoon of olive oil,

1 teaspoon of olive oil,

1 tablespoon of Dijon mustard

1/4 tablespoon of garlic powder

How to Prepare:

Combine all in a bowl. Blend well with a whisk.
Chill overnight to blend flavors.

Easy Cole Slaw

Serves: 1

Carbs Per Serving: 3 to 5

Prep Time: 10 minutes

Effort: Easy

Ingredients:

 raw cabbage (shredded),

mayonnaise, white distilled vinegar salt & pepper (to taste)

How to Prepare:

Per 1 cup of shredded cabbage mix the following:

2 tablespoons of mayonnaise,

2 teaspoons of vinegar, salt & pepper to taste

Easy Egg Plant Salad

Carbs per Serving: 15g total

Effort: Easy

Ingredients:

1 large eggplant – cut 1/2" pieces,

1 large onion – cut 1/2" pieces, (red, white, yellow, Spanish)

1 can pitted black olives – diced small,

1 small jar of Spanish olives diced into small pieces,

1/4 cup of cider vinegar – more to taste,

1 quart tomato sauce – whatever low carb brand you use

How to Prepare:

Mix all chopped ingredients and add the vinegar. Toss well to mix the vinegar with the mixed veggies. Let set a few minutes and toss again. Add the tomato sauce and mix again. Add red pepper and black to taste (1/2 tsp red is hot).

Mix one more time before placing in a 4 ⍰t. Corning ware pot. Bake in the oven at 325`F for about 1 hour

(1 1⁄2 hours is mushy)

Let cool to room temperature, toss and refrigerate before serving (sandwich spread, appetizer, main course with chicken, pork beef).

Suggestions: prep time on the above recipe is about 15 minutes, has a very uni⍰ue taste that satisfies the appetite.

French Dressing 2

Carbs per Serving: 9g total

Effort: Easy

Ingredients: 1⁄2 cup salad oil,

1/3 cup of red wine vinegar,

1 tablespoon of lemon juice,

1 teaspoon of Worcestershire sauce,

1⁄2 teaspoon of salt,

1/4 package of artificial sweetener – to taste,

1/2 teaspoon of dry mustard

1/2 teaspoon of pepper,

1 clove of garlic – minced

How to Prepare:

Put everything in a jar with screw on lid and shake well. Makes about 1 cup

French Dressing

Serves: 4 to 6 servings Carbs Per Serving: very low

Prep Time: 5 minutes Effort: Easy

Ingredients:

1/2 cup of Walden farms ketchup,

1/2 cup of oil (canola or vegetable) ,

1/4 cup of white vinegar,

1 packet of e▢ual,

1 teaspoon of lemon juice dash of pepper

How to Prepare:

stir all ingredients until combined

Cajun Chicken Caesar Salad

Carbs per Serving: 4g total

Effort: Easy

Ingredients:

1 large chicken breast, Cajun spice or cayenne pepper to taste,

2 tablespoons of Hot Sauce,

2 Cups of romaine lettuce,

2 tablespoons of Caesar dressing,

2 tablespoons of parmesan cheese.

How to Prepare:

Sprinkle spices on chicken breast. May be grill on the BBQ, baked, fried, etc. Cut in to 1 inch cubes and toss with hot sauce. Set aside.

Mix lettuce, dressing and cheese. Put on a plate and top with chicken. Top with additional parmesan cheese if desired.

I like mine really hot and spicy so I use cayenne Cajun spice will make it a little milder.

Cottage Cheese Casserole

Carbs per serving: 36g total

Effort: Easy

Ingredients:

3 eggs, slightly beaten

3 cups of cottage cheese small diced onion black pepper to taste

How to Prepare:

Mix all ingredients and pour into a casserole dish. Bake at 350 degrees for 45-50 minutes, or until firm and pulls away from the sides of the pan. Serve warm.

Cranberry Relish

Carbs Pe rServing: 74g total

Effort: Easy

Ingredients:

1 cup of dark rum

1 teaspoon of lemon rind – grated

3⁄4 cup of artificial sweetener (note: can use sugar)

3⁄4 to 1/2 cup odf walnuts – chopped, pecans or almonds

4 cups of cranberries – raw fresh or frozen

How to Prepare:

Put Splenda and rum in saucepan, heat to boiling. Add cranberries & lemon zest, bring back to boil & immediately lower heat so the mixture is on a low, rolling boil, just above a simmer. Cover and cook for 10 minutes, stirring occasionally. Add chopped nuts, mixing in thoroughly Let cook 1-2 min, then remove from heat, cover and let cool completely. The rum & lemon zest add tremendous richness complexity to the sauce. But, if you want to forego the rum, just substitute an eꞎual amount of water.

Double Cranberry Salad

Serves: 8

Carbs per Serving: 3.125g Effort: Easy

Ingredients

2 1⁄2 cups of Diet Iced Botanicals (Cranberry-Raspberry)

1 large package Cranberry Jell-O,

1⁄2 cup of chopped celery,

1/2 cup of chopped pecans,

1 1⁄2 cups of cottage cheese,

1/8 cup of mayonnaise

How to Prepare:

Bring Botanicals to boil. Stir in Jell-O until dissolved. Chill until partially set (thickened –but not solid Pour 1⁄2 in 8x8x2 inch glass pan. Stir 1⁄2 cup celery & 1⁄2 cup nuts into pan—add additional celery & nuts to remaining Jello. Chill 8x8 pan & remaining Jell-O mixture---until Jell-O is firm.Mix together cottage cheese & Mayo---place on top of 8x8 layer of Jell-O. Take remaining Jell-O (if it is firm warm slightly in microwave & pour over cottage cheese).Chill until firm. Cut into 8 servings.

Fancy Pea Salad

Carbs Per Serving: 78g total

Effort: Easy

Ingredients:

2 cups of peas, canned – fancy,

1 1/2 cups of finely chopped onion,

1 cup of celery – chopped

2 cups of lettuce – cut bite-sized,

1 cup of mayonnaise,

10 slices of bacon – cooked and crumbled

1/4 cup of Parmesan cheese

How to Prepare:

Toss peas, onion, celery, and lettuce with mayonnaise in a serving bowl. Sprinkle bacon on top. Sprinkle with Parmesan cheese. Cover; refrigerate overnight.

Little peas, celery, and bacon add crunch and color to this salad. It's a very nice change of pace for a picnic or potluck. Note that you can use frozen peas, if you prefer. You can use whatever variety of lettuce suits your taste. Serves 4-6.

French Dressing

Serves: 4 to 6 servings

Carbs Per Serving: very low

Prep Time: 5 minutes   Effort: Easy

Ingredients:

1⁄2 cup of ketchup,

1⁄2 cup of oil (canola or vegetable)

1⁄4 cup of white vinegar,

1 packet equal,

1 teaspoon of lemon juice dash of pepper

How to Prepare:

stir all ingredients until combined

Ginger Salad Dressing

Serves: 6

Carbs Pe rServing: 1.83g Effort: Easy

Ingredients:

1⁄4 cup of chopped onion,

1⁄4 cup of peanut oil,

Wine vinegar 2 tablespoons,

Water 1 tablespoon,

Ginger root – chopped,

1 tablespoon of chopped celery,

1 tablespoon of soy sauce,

1 1⁄2 teaspoons of tomato paste,

1 1⁄2 teaspoons of splenda,

1 teaspoon of lemon juice,

1 Dash, salt and pepper

How to Prepare:

Combine all ingredients in blender container or wok bowl of food processor fitted with steel knife; process until almost smooth. May be kept refrigerated up to one week.

Grilled Chicken Salad

Carbs per Serving: 31g

 Total Effort: Easy

Ingredients:

1⁄4 cup soy sauce,

1⁄4 cup olive oil,

2 pounds skinless boneless chicken breast – cut in bite size chunks,

Garlic powder – to taste,

2 cups of lettuce,

1 large tomato,

1 medium cucumber,

1⁄2 red onion black pepper – to taste balsamic vinegar – to taste

How to Prepare:

Heat oil in non-stick fry pan Saute chicken with garlic powder until just starting to turn a golden brown. Add soy sauce. Simmer on low heat for about 5 to 10 minutes. The oil will float a little to the top. That's okay. Make salad with the remaining items. Sprinkle with black pepper. NO SALT! That's what the soy sauce is for. When salad is ready, pour the hot mixture of chicken, oil and soy onto the salad. Add balsamic vinegar to taste and toss. The lettuce will wilt a little. You will love it!

Honey Mustard!

Serves: One

Carbs per Serving: About 3

Prep Time: Less than one minute!

Effort: Easy

 Ingredients:

1 Tbs. of Dijion Mustard,

1 Tbs. Spicey Brown Mustard,

2 Tbs. low fat Heavy Whipping Cream,

1 Packet Splenda

How to Prepare:

Mix all ingredients and serve! Origionally, I thought this up as a dip for chicken, but it also makes the BEST salad dressing. If you've been missing honey mustard dressing

Hot Chinese Chicken Salad

Carbs Per Serving: no counts provided

Effort: Easy

Ingredients:

For two large salads:

2 chicken breast – cooked with desired seasoning,

2 large bowls of lettuce,

Tomatoes (optional) for Gout diets keep the amount of tomatoes at a minimum, Crumbled bacon (optional), Hot peppers (optional) Slivered almonds (optional), Desired shredded cheese (Cheddar is excellent)

Dressing (The Best Part):

1⁄2 cup oil,

1/3 cup apple cider vinegar,

1 Tablespoon soy sauce (low sodium),

2 packets E?ual – Splenda

1 Dash ginger,

1 Dash pepper,

1 Dash garlic salt

How to Prepare:

Bring ingredients of dressing to a boil in a pan and stir with Wisk. Once all ingredients are well-blended, pour over salads.

Hot German Turnip Salad

Carbs per Serving: 4g

Total Effort :Easy

Ingredients:

1 cup mayonnaise,

3 Tablespoons white wine,

2 teaspoons vinegar,

1⁄2 cup bacon grease,

1⁄2 teaspoon fresh dill,

2 packages artificial sweetener – sweet n low,

3⁄4 teaspoon salt,

1/8 teaspoon pepper bacon strips – crushed

2 teaspoons onion

How to Prepare:

Whisk all ingredients together. Makes about 2 cups. Use about 1⁄4 to 1⁄2 cup per large turnip, boiled until soft. Add crushed bacon and 2 tablespoons onion sauted in bacon grease.